Genomics

Editors

JOHN DUSTIN LOY
JESSICA L. KLABNIK
NIAL J. O'BOYLE

VETERINARY CLINICS
OF NORTH AMERICA:
FOOD ANIMAL PRACTICE

www.vetfood.theclinics.com

Consulting Editor
ROBERT A. SMITH

November 2024 • Volume 40 • Number 3

ELSEVIER

1600 John F. Kennedy Boulevard • Suite 1800 • Philadelphia, Pennsylvania, 19103-2899

http://www.vetfood.theclinics.com

VETERINARY CLINICS OF NORTH AMERICA: FOOD ANIMAL PRACTICE Volume 40, Number 3
November 2024 ISSN 0749-0720, ISBN-13: 978-0-443-12965-0

Editor: Taylor Hayes
Developmental Editor: Varun Gopal

Veterinary Clinics of North America: Food Animal Practice (ISSN 0749-0720) is published in March, July, and November by Elsevier Inc., 360 Park Avenue South, New York, NY 10010-1710. Subscription prices are $281.00 per year (domestic individuals), $100.00 per year (domestic students/residents), $298.00 per year (Canadian individuals), $356.00 per year (international individuals) $100.00 per year (Canadian students), and $165.00 (international students). For institutional access pricing please contact Customer Service via the contact information below. To receive student/resident rate, orders must be accompanied by name of affiliated institution, date of term, and the signature of program/residency coordinator on institution letterhead. *Clinics* subscription prices. All prices are subject to change without notice. Orders, claims, and journal inquiries: Please visit our Support Hub page https://service.elsevier.com for assistance.

Reprints. For copies of 100 or more, of articles in this publication, please contact the Commercial Reprints Department, Elsevier Inc., 360 Park Avenue South, New York, NY 10010-1710. Tel.: 212-633-3874; Fax: 212-633-3820; E-mail: reprints@elsevier.com.

Veterinary Clinics of North America: Food Animal Practice is covered in *Current Contents/Agriculture, Biology and Environmental Sciences, MEDLINE/PubMed (Index Medicus), and Excerpta Medica.*

Contributors

CONSULTING EDITOR

ROBERT A. SMITH, DVM, MS
Diplomate, American Board of Veterinary Practitioners; Veterinary Research and Consulting Services, LLC, Greeley, Colorado, USA

EDITORS

JOHN DUSTIN LOY, DVM, PhD
Diplomate of the American College of Veterinary Microbiologists; Professor and Director, Nebraska Veterinary Diagnostic Center, School of Veterinary Medicine and Biomedical Sciences, University of Nebraska-Lincoln, Lincoln, Nebraska, USA

JESSICA L. KLABNIK, DVM, MPH, PhD
Diplomate of the American College of Theriogenologists; Assistant Professor of Theriogenology, Department of Clinical Sciences, Auburn University College of Veterinary Medicine, Auburn, Alabama, USA

NIAL J. O'BOYLE, BVSc, MS, MBA, MRCVS
School of Veterinary Medicine and Science, University of Nottingham, Sutton Bonington Campus, Leicestershire, United Kingdom

AUTHORS

PRIYANKA BANERJEE, PhD
Postdoctoral Researcher, Department of Animal Sciences, Auburn University, Auburn, Alabama, USA

DONAGH P. BERRY, PhD, MSc Bioinformatics, BAgr, Sc, BSc
Geneticist, Animal & Grassland Research and Innovation Centre, Teagasc, Moorepark, Cork, Ireland

MIKE COFFEY, PhD
Professor, Livestock Informatics, Animal Breeding and Genomics Team, SRUC – Scotland's Rural College, Edinburgh, United Kingdom

PATRICK M.R. COMYN, DVM
Owner, Virginia Herd Health Management Service P.C, Madison, Virginia, USA

JAMIE T. COURTER, PhD
State Beef Genetics Extension Specialist, Division of Animal Sciences, University of Missouri, Columbia, Missouri, USA

WELLISON J.S. DINIZ, PhD
Assistant Professor, Department of Animal Sciences, Auburn University, Auburn, Alabama, USA

KIM EGAN, DVM, MBA
Director of Technical Service, Genex Cooperative, Shawano, Wisconsin, USA

SUSANNE HINKLEY, DVM, PhD
Director, Clinical Diagnostics, Neogen Genomics, Lincoln, Nebraska, USA

JESSICA L. KLABNIK, DVM, MPH, PhD
Diplomate of the American College of Theriogenologists; Assistant Professor of Theriogenology, Department of Clinical Sciences, Auburn University College of Veterinary Medicine, Auburn, Alabama, USA

JOHN DUSTIN LOY, DVM, PhD
Diplomate of the American College of Veterinary Microbiologists; Professor and Director, Nebraska Veterinary Diagnostic Center, School of Veterinary Medicine and Biomedical Sciences, University of Nebraska-Lincoln, Lincoln, Nebraska, USA

RAPHAEL MRODE, PhD
Professor, Livestock Informatics, Animal Breeding and Genomics Team, SRUC – Scotland's Rural College, Edinburgh, United Kingdom

MACI L. MUELLER, PhD
Assistant Professor, Department of Animal Sciences and Industry, Kansas State University, Manhattan, Kansas, USA

NIAL J. O'BOYLE, BVSc, MS, MBA, MRCVS
School of Veterinary Medicine and Science, University of Nottingham, Sutton Bonington Campus, Leicestershire, United Kingdom

TROY N. ROWAN, PhD
Assistant Professor, Departments of Animal Science and Large Animal Clinical Sciences, University of Tennessee, Knoxville, Tennessee, USA

MATTHEW L. SPANGLER, PhD, MSc, BSc (Anim Sci)
Professor, Department of Animal Science, University of Nebraska-Lincoln, Lincoln, Nebraska, USA

RANDALL SPARE, DVM
Veterinarian, Ashland Veterinary Center Inc., Ashland, Kansas, USA

RICHARD G. TAIT Jr, MS, PhD, PAS
Director, Genetics Product Development, Neogen Genomics, Lincoln, Nebraska, USA

MARCO WINTERS, MSc
Head of Animal Genetics, AHDB - Agriculture and Horticulture Development Board, Coventry, United Kingdom

Contents

Genetic mutations, both favorable and unfavorable, are the raw material for improvement in livestock populations. The random inheritance of these mutations is essential for generating progenies with genetic potential greater than their parents. These mutations can act either in a simple manner, such that a single alteration disrupts phenotype, or in a complex manner where hundreds or thousands of mutations of small effect create a continuous distribution of phenotypes. Selection tools leverage phenotypic records, pedigrees, and genomics to estimate the genetic potential of individual animals. This more accurate accounting of genetic potential has generated enormous gains in livestock populations.

Genetic evaluations in beef cattle have evolved over the past 50 years relative to the hardware or software used, the statistical methodology underpinning them, and the traits evaluated. However, the underlying premise has remained the same; to generate predictions of genetic merit such that selection decisions can be made that materialize as phenotypic changes in commercial animals. The wide-spread availability and adoption of genomic technology has enabled more accurate genetic predictions of young animals albeit with the requirement of continual collection and reporting of phenotypic data.

In the evolving landscape of beef cattle management, veterinarians are transitioning from their traditional role of treating diseases to becoming proactive advisors. This article explores how veterinarians with knowledge of genetic tools are poised to be vital in addressing the fundamental industry challenges. It highlights the role of genetic selection in reducing calving difficulties, emphasizing its benefits for animal health and welfare. The article also surveys the genomic technologies available and discusses the importance of integrating these insights with veterinary expertise to support informed decisions in selection, mating, and marketing strategies.

cradle to the grave as well as parentage discovery. The information available per animal aids more informed breeding and management decisions, including mating advice, and determining the optimal role and eventual fate of each animal.

The US beef and dairy industries have made remarkable advances in sustainability and productivity through technological advancements, including selective breeding. Yet, challenges persist due to the complex nature of quantitative traits. While the beef industry has progressed in adopting genomic technologies, the availability of phenotypic data remains an obstacle. To meet the need for sustainable production systems, novel traits are being targeted for selection. Additionally, emerging approaches such as genome editing and high-throughput phenotyping hold promise for further genetic progress. Future research should address the challenges of translating functional genomic findings into practical applications, while simultaneously harnessing analytical methods.

The current article is a forward-looking synopsis to provide insights into the current state of the industry and some areas where future work may hold additional promise. The integration of genomics into the dairy and beef industries is multifaceted and will impact production gains, identification and management of genetic diseases, and streamlined breeding and selection approaches. Veterinarians are uniquely poised to educate clients, integrate genomic data with existing metrics, and assist in decision-making that will impact the future shape of the global herd.

VETERINARY CLINICS OF NORTH AMERICA: FOOD ANIMAL PRACTICE

Preface

Genomics for the Modern Beef and Dairy Practitioner

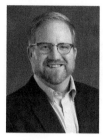
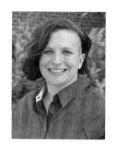
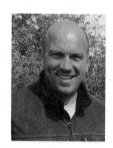

John Dustin Loy,
DVM, PhD, DACVM

Jessica L. Klabnik, DVM,
MPH, PhD, DACT
Editors

Nial J. O'Boyle, BVSc,
MS, MBA, MRCVS

Genomics continues to increase in the scope of applications resulting in subsequent demand for ruminant production industries. Veterinary practitioners play a crucial role in aiding in the implementation of genomic strategies on the farm. Following successful application of these technologies, the resulting increases in animal health and welfare can ultimately increase production efficiency, farm economics, and animal well-being. In the article in this issue by Rowan, "Genetics and Genomics 101," fundamental background information is presented to solidify core concepts that are critical for veterinarians to provide appropriate consultation. Genomics can be used in the beef industry for both genetic evaluations ("Beef Genetic Evaluations" by Spangler and Berry) and modern approaches to medicine and welfare ("Innovating Beef Cattle Veterinary Practices: Leveraging Genetic and Genomic Tools" by Mueller and colleagues). Proper sampling and laboratory considerations for successful genomic testing are outlined in "Sampling and Laboratory Logistics: How to Collect DNA Samples and Overview of Techniques for Laboratory Analysis" by Hinkley and Tait. Practitioners can impact both dairy and beef industries by consulting on genetic and genomic strategies across a broad range of producer goals and needs ("The Private Practitioner: A Veterinary Practitioner's Perspective to the Application of Bovine Genomics in Client Herds" by Comyn); this ultimately affects economics of both the farm and industry ("Role of Veterinary Practitioners in the Genomic Era in Dairy: Economic Impact" by Egan). Although *Veterinary Clinics of North America: Food Animal Practice* focuses on regional needs, cattle production industries are global, and methods of applications and lessons learned are informative worldwide. "European Dairy Cattle Evaluations and International Use of Genomic Data" by Winters and colleagues discusses the European dairy cattle evaluations and the international use and application of genomic data. As the beef and dairy industries move forward, both in North America

Vet Clin Food Anim 40 (2024) ix–x
https://doi.org/10.1016/j.cvfa.2024.06.001
0749-0720/24/© 2024 Published by Elsevier Inc.

and globally, a national genomic testing scheme would both benefit producers and allow for research and industry progress to develop more efficiently and effectively ("The Benefit of a National Genomic Testing Scheme" by Berry and Spangler). Looking forward, novel genomic technologies will allow for advances in animal health and production that have not been greatly impacted by traditional breeding schemes ("Advancing Dairy and Beef Genetics Through Genomic Technologies" by Banerjee and Diniz). The final article, "Future Directions for Ruminant Genomics" by Klabnik and colleagues, is a forward-looking synopsis to provide insights into the current state of the industry and some areas where future work may hold additional promise. Overall, the integration of genomics into the dairy and beef industries is multifaceted and will impact production gains and economic efficiencies, allow for rapid identification and management of genetic diseases, improve cattle health and well-being, and result in more streamlined breeding and selection approaches. Veterinarians can offer invaluable guidance in applying genomic data to assist producers in improving productivity, health, and economic returns because of their expertise in herd health, genetics, and management, which is the focus of this special issue.

DISCLOSURES

The authors have nothing to disclose.

John Dustin Loy, DVM, PhD, DACVM
Nebraska Veterinary Diagnostic Center
School of Veterinary Medicine and
Biomedical Sciences
University of Nebraska–Lincoln
115B NVDC, 4040 East Campus Loop North
Lincoln, NE 68583-0907, USA

Jessica L. Klabnik, DVM, MPH, PhD, DACT
Department of Clinical Sciences
College of Veterinary Medicine
1500 Wire Road
Auburn, AL 36830, USA

Nial J. O'Boyle, BVSc, MS, MBA, MRCVS
School of Veterinary Medicine and Science
University of Nottingham
Sutton Bonington Campus
Leicestershire LE12 5RD, UK

E-mail addresses:
jdloy@unl.edu (J.D. Loy)
jlk0066@auburn.edu (J.L. Klabnik)
nialjoboyle@gmail.com (N.J. O'Boyle)

Genetics and Genomics 101

Troy N. Rowan, PhD[a,b,*]

KEYWORDS

- Cattle • Genomics • DNA • Breeding • Complex traits • Genotype

KEY POINTS

- Animal breeders leverage the random inheritance of deoxyribose nucleic acid to genetically improve animal populations.
- The rate of genetic progress is a function of selection intensity, selection accuracy, the amount of trait-associated genetic variation, and the generation interval.
- Innovations in genetic prediction allow for more accurate selection of younger animals, driving significant genetic progress.
- Genomic testing has accelerated genetic gain across the beef and dairy industries.

INTRODUCTION

Humans have been selectively breeding and improving cattle since domestication in the Fertile Crescent nearly 10,000 years ago.[1] Our methods for selecting animals and amplifying elite genetics have changed enormously since then. Still, the core concepts that breeders exploit have mostly remained the same: identify animals that received a favorable sampling of parental genetics and use them as parents in the subsequent generation. Our methods for identifying genetically superior animals have become more accurate as we have gained a more detailed understanding of genetic inheritance patterns and developed methods for tracking them across generations. This has resulted in a transition from selection based on purely visual characteristics to selection on more accurately measured phenotypes to estimates of genetic merit to genetic merit estimates informed by genomics.

This review will briefly introduce the underlying concepts enabling genetic selection for complex traits in beef cattle. It reviews basic molecular genetics concepts, inheritance patterns, complex and Mendelian traits, heritability, and genetic prediction.

[a] Department of Animal Science, University of Tennessee, 2506 River Drive, Knoxville, TN 37996, USA; [b] Department Large Animal Clinical Sciences, University of Tennessee, Knoxville, TN, USA
* Department of Animal Science, University of Tennessee, 2506 River Drive, Knoxville, TN 37996.
E-mail address: trowan@utk.edu
Twitter: @TroyNRowan (T.N.R.)

Vet Clin Food Anim 40 (2024) 345–355
https://doi.org/10.1016/j.cvfa.2024.05.001
0749-0720/24/© 2024 Elsevier Inc. All rights reserved, including those for text and data mining, AI training, and similar technologies.
vetfood.theclinics.com

A CRASH COURSE ON THE GENOME

As with all living things, deoxyribose nucleic acid (DNA) serves as a biological blueprint for the development, growth, and physiologic abilities of cattle. The total DNA content of an individual is referred to as the genome. The cattle genome consists of around 2.6 billion base pairs of nucleotides spread across 30 pairs of chromosomes, including the sex chromosomes X and Y.[2] Chromosomes are the physical structures that DNA organizes itself into within the nucleus of cells. Like nearly all mammals, cattle have 2 sets of chromosomes, one inherited from each parent at fertilization.

A relatively minor proportion (<2%) of the nucleotide content differs among cattle.[3] This small variable minority of the genome drives the heritable differences among animals. These variations occur as mutations caused by imperfect DNA replication machinery, occasionally making errors when copying DNA during mitosis (somatic) and meiosis (germline).[4,5] Somatic mutations do not contribute to genetic variation between individuals as they are not passed from parents to offspring. Germline mutations in the gonads will be passed onto offspring produced by mutated gametes. These mutations serve as the raw material for all genetic variation among animals. In cattle, mutations occur once every 100,000,000 base pairs. As such, every gamete is expected to contain at least 30 de novo mutations.[6] Mutations can manifest in a variety of ways. The most common are single nucleotide polymorphisms (SNPs), where a single base pair is mutated at a given location (locus) in the genome. Small mutations resulting in multiple base pairs being inserted or deleted from the original genome are called indels.[7] Mutations that cause more extensive structural rearrangements of the genome that severely interrupt gene function can also occur.[8] Due to the complexity of structural variation, most current commercially available genomic technologies observe only SNPs and indels.

Our more practical interest in genetics in animal breeding is understanding its effects in shaping economically relevant phenotypes. This link between genetic mutations and end phenotype requires multiple intermediate functions and features. The 2.6 billion base pairs in the cattle genome contain around 30,000 features known as genes.[2] While the basic unit of inheritance is colloquially termed a gene, a more biologically rooted definition is the portion of the genome that encodes a protein or other functional molecule.

Multiple molecular intermediates link genotype to phenotypic variation. DNA is typically wrapped around proteins called histones that are further arranged into structures called chromatin when not in use.[9] In specific environmental and development contexts, gene regions of DNA become accessible to the cellular machinery that reads genic DNA and synthesizes ribonucleic acid (RNA) in the process of transcription. These "expressed" genes can then be modified or spliced before the final messenger RNA (mRNA) is decoded by ribosomes into polypeptides that come together to form proteins that go on to carry out the biological functions that ultimately result in phenotypes.[10]

GENETIC INHERITANCE: MENDELIAN AND COMPLEX TRAITS

The ability to select genetically superior animals relies on patterns of genetic inheritance shared across sexually reproducing organisms. During the final stages of oocyte and sperm development, meiosis reduces the number of chromosomes in half, making these cells 1N. After fertilization, this results in a diploid (ie, 2N) embryo that has inherited a random half of each of its parent's genomes.[11] This random combination of parental chromosomes, combined with recombination that occurs during crossing-over events, is responsible for generating substantial amounts of variation in the inherited genetics, even by full siblings.

Genetic inheritance is most easily understood at the level of a single locus. At a locus with an A and B mutation (allele), a heterozygous parent (AB) has a 50% chance of passing either allele to an offspring. This means that a mating of heterozygous parents will, on average, produce offspring that are 25% AA, 50% AB, and 25% BB. At heterozygous sites, inheritance is effectively a coin flip as to which allele will be passed on to offspring.

Traits can be broken into 2 major classes based on their complexity: Both in the number of genetic loci that impact phenotype and how those variants act. We refer to this complexity as a trait's genetic architecture.[12] Traits with simple (Mendelian or monogenic) inheritance patterns are driven by a single or very small number of mutations. In contrast, complex traits are affected by hundreds or thousands of mutations spread throughout the genome.[13] Mutations can act additively (heterozygous genotype has an effect that is the midpoint between opposite homozygotes), dominantly (the effect of one allele wholly or partially masks the effect of the other), or epistatically (the effect of an allele is affected by the genotype at another locus).[14]

Some Mendelian traits are essential in livestock breeding contexts. Most of these mutant phenotypes are either dominant (one copy of the mutant allele results in phenotypic change) or recessive (2 copies of the mutant allele alter phenotype). Traits such as polledness,[15] black coat color,[16] and various congenital genetic defects[17] demonstrate Mendelian inheritance patterns. With simple traits, knowledge of inheritance patterns and parental genotypes can accurately predict the proportions of offspring genotypes and phenotypes. Genetic tests for these mutations have allowed breeders to manage recessive defects by avoiding mating characters rather than culling carrier animals.[18]

COMPLEX TRAIT INHERITANCE AND HERITABILITY

Most economically relevant traits in beef and dairy cattle are complex, driven by hundreds or thousands of causal mutations of relatively small effect spread throughout the genome.[19] The causal mechanisms of these mutations can be quite diverse. Mutations within genes can disrupt or alter the functionality of the gene's ultimate protein product.[20] Other mutations that occur in regulatory regions outside of genes can alter the level of expression, posttranslational splicing, or epigenetic modifications, resulting in different abundances or versions of mRNA.[21] These mutations ultimately result in altered biological function that affects an animal's phenotype. Compared with Mendelian traits, complex traits are more difficult to predict from knowledge of parental phenotypes. The random inheritance of thousands of small effect alleles makes the distribution of possible phenotypes quite large.

When offspring inherit half of their parental genetic material, they inherit half of their genetic potential for a trait. This inheritance leads to a clear resemblance between parent and offspring, the degree to which is referred to as heritability. Heritability is the proportion of phenotypic variation that can be attributed to genetic variation. The 2 main types of heritability can be broken into broad sense ($H^2 = \sigma_G^2/\sigma_P^2$), where σ_G^2 is all genetic variance (additive, dominance, and epistasis), and narrow sense ($H^2 = \sigma_A^2/\sigma_P^2$), where σ_A^2 is the additive genetic variance.[22] For applications in breeding, we typically restrict our discussion of heritability to the narrow sense value, as the additive genetic variance is the primary driver of resemblance between relatives.[23]

It is important to note that heritabilities are statistical, not biological properties, and are a function of the population in which genetic and phenotypic variance components are estimated. Reductions in environmental variation due to management interventions can increase the relative proportion of a trait driven by genetic factors. Heritabilities of economically important traits in cattle range from around 0.60 (stature) to 0.10 (fertility; American Angus Association & American Holstein Association). It is important to note that even the most highly heritable phenotypes are still affected by environmental factors. Examples of heritabilities for economically relevant traits in Holstein and Angus cattle are shown in **Table 1**.

The random inheritance of parental genomes that leads to genetic variation among siblings is called Mendelian sampling (**Fig. 1**). In traits affected by many mutations, the random sampling of alleles from parents results in normally distributed, continuous offspring phenotypes.[24] Siblings will resemble their parents and each other, but variation in genetic merit will exist on either side of the parental average. Animal breeding exploits this variation to drive genetic improvement by selecting individuals better than their parents' average.[25] Without Mendelian sampling, genetic progress through breeding would be impossible, as all offspring would be the same quality as their parental generation.

GENETIC PROGRESS AND THE BREEDER'S EQUATION

Selection decisions in breeding programs rely on identifying animals that received favorable samples of parental genetics. The rate at which a population or herd makes genetic change (ΔG) is central to the success of a breeding program.[26] We can determine the rate of ΔG using the breeder's equation. In this case, $\Delta G = \dfrac{i \; r_{BV,\widehat{BV}} \; \sigma_A}{L}$, where i is the intensity of selection (the proportion of animals that go on to become parents in the next generation), $r_{BV,\widehat{BV}}$ is the accuracy of selection (correlation between an animal's true genetic merit, BV, and the selection metric, $\widehat{BV}$), σ_A is the amount of genetic variation in the population for the trait of interest, and L is the generation interval (average age of parents in the population).[27] Shifts in any of these values will alter the rate of ΔG.

Selection intensity is the difference between selected animals and the population's average before selection. When fewer individuals are chosen to be parents, this gap grows. One of the main ways that selection intensity has been altered in cattle breeding scenarios is through artificial insemination and embryo transfer.[28] This has allowed fewer bulls and cows to serve as parents in the seedstock programs that drive genetic progress in their elite populations and commercial herds. In commercial beef herds, bulls produce more calves per year than cows (often 25–35 times as many).

Table 1
Heritabilities of assorted economically relevant traits in American Angus and Holstein populations

Trait	Breed	H²	Trait	Breed	H²
Calving ease[a]	Angus	0.19	Calving ease[b]	Holstein	0.07
Weaning weight[a]	Angus	0.28	Somatic cell count[b]	Holstein	0.12
Heifer pregnancy[a]	Angus	0.15	Heifer conception rate[b]	Holstein	0.01
Mature weight[a]	Angus	0.35	Productive life[b]	Holstein	0.08
Mature height[a]	Angus	0.59	Stature[c]	Holstein	0.58
Docility[a]	Angus	0.44	Milk yield[b]	Holstein	0.20
Marbling[a]	Angus	0.48	Fat yield[b]	Holstein	0.20
Carcass weight[a]	Angus	0.44	Protein Yield[b]	Holstein	0.20

[a] From American Angus Association: https://www.angus.org/Nce/Heritabilities.
[b] From Council on Dairy Cattle Breeding: https://uscdcb.com/individual-traits/.
[c] From Holstein USA: https://www.holsteinusa.com/genetic_evaluations/ss_linear.html.

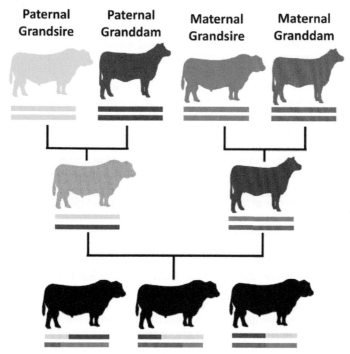

Paternal Grandsire **Paternal Granddam** **Maternal Grandsire** **Maternal Granddam**

Fig. 1. An example of Mendelian sampling. This represents a 3 generation pedigree for 3 full-sibling brothers. Each animal receives 50% of their DNA from each parent. However, the 50% they receive is random. This results in deviations from the expectation that they share 25% of their DNA with each grandparent.

This increased selection intensity means that most genetic progress in commercial herds comes from bull purchases rather than replacement heifer selection decisions.[29] Sufficient trait-associated genetic variation must also exist in a trait for genetic progress to be possible. Without genetic variation between individuals, matings cannot generate different selection responses.[30]

The 2 chief drivers of genetic progress in livestock breeding programs are selection accuracy and generation interval.[31] Selection accuracy is the correlation between a selection metric and an animal's true genetic merit (ie, breeding value).[32] When selecting based on phenotypes, the selection accuracy equals a trait's heritability. As a result, phenotypic selection on more highly heritable traits can generate genetic gain more rapidly than those that are lowly heritable. It is easier to think of selection accuracy as how often the "correct animal" (ie, the one with superior true genetic potential) is selected. Selection tools based on statistical estimates of an animal's genetic merit are more accurate than selecting on phenotype alone. Consequently, animal breeding research has focused on strategies for estimating animals' breeding values based on phenotypic, familial relationships, and, more recently, genomics.[33,34] Ultimately, these tools aim to identify animals that received favorable samples of parental genomes before observing their offspring's performance.

ESTIMATES OF GENETIC POTENTIAL

We can never know an animal's true breeding value or genetic potential with absolute certainty, so we are left to statistically estimate it using various sources of information.

These statistical estimates of an animal's genetic potential are called estimated breeding values (EBVs).[35] In the context of the breeder's equation, EBVs can accelerate the rate of genetic gain both by improving selection accuracy and reducing the generation interval.[31] EBVs perform 2 main functions: First, they control for environmental and management differences between herds that might affect animal phenotypes, and further, they estimate which genetics an individual inherited from its parents (ie, Mendelian sampling, see **Fig. 1**). This leads to more accurate estimates of genetic merit earlier in an animal's life. This includes increased selection accuracy for traits not expressed until later in an animal's life, such as longevity or sustained fertility.[36] When paired with advanced reproductive technologies like artificial insemination, embryo transfer, and in vitro fertilization, this allows superior genetics to be amplified while an animal is young, resulting in vast improvements in generation interval.[37]

Phenotypic recording is at the core of generating accurate genetic predictions.[38,39] Estimates of breeding values are calculated via linear mixed models through the best linear unbiased prediction (BLUP) method.[33,40] In the BLUP model, fixed effects account for environmental and other nongenic factors that alter phenotypes. Contemporary groups are commonly used to account for farm-by-farm variation in management and environment. Groups are formed based on a combination of shared herds, years, and seasons in which animals are raised.[41,42] Without sufficient numbers of phenotypes recorded across many contemporary groups, EBV calculation is impossible.[43,44] Consequently, as phenotypic datasets grow, the accuracy with which EBVs predict an animal's genetic merit also increases.

More accurately accounting for relationships between individuals in an evaluation can help increase the quality of predictions.[45] This has traditionally been accomplished using pedigrees. Pedigree-based genetic evaluations use assumed coefficients of relationship.[46,47] Inaccurate pedigrees caused by incorrect parentage identification can degrade the quality of genetic predictions.[48] Historically, adding progeny records to a genetic evaluation was the most critical contributor to improved EBV accuracies.

In beef and dairy populations, the calculation of EBVs is typically performed by breed associations or other third-party organizations that aggregate phenotypic and pedigree data. The US dairy industry relies on the Council on Dairy Cattle Breeding (Bowie, MD) to calculate EBVs for over 50 traits.[49] Some dairy breeds opt to calculate genetic predictions for certain traits within breed (eg, Holstein type traits). Beef cattle genetic evaluations are generally performed by individual breed associations, though some breeds have leveraged genetic connectedness to run multibreed evaluations (eg, International Genetics Solutions).[50] Breed associations are typically responsible for registration, maintaining pedigrees, phenotypic recording, and, more recently, managing DNA sample repositories.

Dairy genetic predictions are reported as predicted transmitting abilities (PTAs), whereas beef cattle predictions are typically reported as estimated progeny differences (EPDs). Both PTAs and EPDs are one-half of an animal's EBV.[51] This division of an EBV by 2 is performed because an animal can only pass half of its genetic material to progeny. This allows a sire and dam's PTA or EPD to be summed to predict an average offspring EBV. An EBV or PTA can be interpreted as the expected difference between the average progeny of 2 different sires when bred to a large set of genetically similar animals. These values are only useful when comparing between selection candidates or a selection candidate relative to the population in which the values are calculated.

Calculating genomic predictions is possible for any heritable trait and for which enough phenotypes have been recorded. In beef cattle populations, easily collected growth traits have been the most heavily recorded and were the first phenotypes to receive EPDs.[43] Similarly, PTAs for milk production and component traits in dairy cattle have been evaluated for decades. Recently, fertility, feed efficiency, sustainability, and other health and disease traits have begun being evaluated in beef[52] and dairy cattle.[53,54] In the future, sensor technologies, computer vision, and automatic milking systems can help generate new high-dimensional phenotypes that allow for genetic evaluations to expand the suite of traits that are evaluated.[55]

GENOMICS AND GENOMIC PREDICTION

The most important development in genetic evaluation since BLUP has been the inclusion of genomics into EBV calculations.[31] Broadly speaking, genomics is the study of how an individual's complete set of DNA works together at the functional level to alter phenotypes. In a breeding context, genomics typically refers to the use of a large set of molecular markers to more accurately predict an animal's EBV.[56] Genomic-enhanced breeding values increase the accuracy of genetic predictions in young, unproven animals before they produce any progeny. As a result, genomic selection alters ΔG by further increasing selection accuracy for young animals, thereby reducing generation interval.[31]

Genomic tests rely on the fact that DNA is inherited in large chunks, called haplotypes, from each parent. Because a statistical relationship exists between the identity of alleles at positions near each other on chromosomes (genetic linkage),[57] a subset of "marker" variants can be used to capture and track large segments of DNA that are likely to be inherited together. This realization led to innovations in the statistical methods used to calculate EBVs. Novel methods include approaches that leverage genome-wide marker data to either estimate the effects of individual segments[34] or to better resolve relationships between individuals rather than assuming pedigree-based relationship coefficients.[58]

Before genomic testing, elite sires, particularly in dairy populations, were identified via progeny test, where promising young bulls were bred to cows and waited until their daughters entered production and had phenotypes recorded to augment their EBVs and inform selection decisions.[59] This system created a massive amount of genetic lag, as the average age of widely used sires was well over 7 years old.[31] With the inclusion of genomics into EBV calculations, the industry was able to rapidly identify genetically elite sires early in life, resulting in massive genetic gain over just a few years. Now, progeny tests are all but a thing of the past, and selection decisions are often made as genomic test results are returned.

Most modern genomic tests leverage the same microarray technology that enabled the first genomic predictions in the late 2000s.[60] These tests use selected subsets of the tens of millions of variants that exist in cattle. Useful markers are those that are (1) SNPs or small indels, (2) evenly spaced (to account for large segments of DNA), and (3) highly variable (can differentiate between individuals). Genotyping arrays typically assay between 20,000 and 100,000 variants throughout the cattle genome. Interestingly, beyond a certain number of markers, current methods fail to produce further increase in accuracy as more are added.[61] That said, emerging methods that explicitly model causal or functional variants show promise in improving genomic predictions.[62] Further, other approaches that leverage direct DNA sequencing have become more practical and potentially cheaper alternatives to array-based genotyping.[63,64]

SUMMARY

Variation between animals is the raw material for genetic progress. Selection for complex traits relies on identifying progeny that received a favorable sampling of their parental genomes. The rate at which genetic progress occurs is a function of selection intensity, selection accuracy, genetic variation, and the average age of parents. Advances in animal breeding have enhanced our ability to accurately select young animals. At the same time, advanced reproductive technologies enabled superior genetics to be amplified across the population. Selection tools in the form of EBVs allow producers to make mating decisions based on statistical predictions of individuals' genetic potential. Further developments in genotyping technology have enabled genomic selection, increasing selection accuracy for young and unproven animals. These innovations and strategies allow the genetic improvement of any complex trait, from growth and performance to fertility to disease resistance to welfare traits.

CLINICS CARE POINTS

- The random sampling of parental genes into gametes is the major driver of genetic differences between relatives and can result in siblings having large differences in genetic merit.
- Economically important traits are under varying degrees of genetic control (heritability). Reproductive and fitness-related traits tend to be less heritable than growth and performance traits.
- Genetic selection tools (EPDs and PTAs) can aid breeders accelerate genetic progress, namely through increasing selection accuracy and decreasing generation intervals.
- Genomic testing in purebred populations increases the accuracy of predictions in unproven animals (ie, those that have not produced any progeny).

DISCLOSURE

The author has nothing to disclose.

FUNDING

USDA-NIFA Grant No. 2022-67015-36214; FFAR Grant No. 22-000087.

REFERENCES

1. Loftus RT, MacHugh DE, Bradley DG, et al. Evidence for two independent domestications of cattle. Proc. Natl. Acad. Sci. U.S.A 1994;91(7):2757–61.
2. Rosen BD, Bickhart DM, Schnabel RD, et al. De novo assembly of the cattle reference genome with single-molecule sequencing. GigaScience 2020;9(3). https://doi.org/10.1093/gigascience/giaa021.
3. Chen N, Fu W, Zhao J, et al. BGVD: An integrated database for bovine sequencing variations and selective signatures. Dev Reprod Biol 2020;18(2):186–93.
4. Veltman JA, Brunner HG. De novo mutations in human genetic disease. Nat Rev Genet 2012;13(8):565–75.
5. Kijas JW, Menzies M, Ingham A. Sequence diversity and rates of molecular evolution between sheep and cattle genes. Anim Genet 2006;37(2):171–4.
6. Charlier C, Li W, Harland C, et al. NGS-based reverse genetic screen for common embryonic lethal mutations compromising fertility in livestock. Genome Res 2016; 26(10):1333–41.
7. Mullaney JM, Mills RE, Pittard WS, et al. Small insertions and deletions (INDELs) in human genomes. Hum Mol Genet 2010;19(R2):R131–6.

8. Gerasimavicius L, Livesey BJ, Marsh JA. Loss-of-function, gain-of-function and dominant-negative mutations have profoundly different effects on protein structure. Nat Commun 2022;13(1):1–15.

9. Klemm SL, Shipony Z, Greenleaf WJ. Chromatin accessibility and the regulatory epigenome. Nat Rev Genet 2019;20(4):207–20.

10. Crick FH. On protein synthesis. Symp Soc Exp Biol 1958;12:138–63.

11. Bolcun-Filas E, Handel MA. Meiosis: the chromosomal foundation of reproduction. Biol Reprod 2018;99(1):112–26.

12. Fu W, O'Connor TD, Akey JM. Genetic architecture of quantitative traits and complex diseases. Curr Opin Genet Dev 2013;23(6):678–83.

13. Barton NH, Etheridge AM, Véber A. The infinitesimal model: Definition, derivation, and implications. Theor Popul Biol 2017;118:50–73.

14. Cordell HJ. Epistasis: what it means, what it doesn't mean, and statistical methods to detect it in humans. Hum Mol Genet 2002;11(20):2463–8.

15. Wiedemar N, Tetens J, Jagannathan V, et al. Independent polled mutations leading to complex gene expression differences in cattle. PLoS One 2014;9(3):e93435.

16. Werth LA, Hawkins GA, Eggen A, et al. Rapid communication: melanocyte stimulating hormone receptor (MC1R) maps to bovine chromosome 18. J Anim Sci 1996;74(1):262.

17. Ciepłoch A, Rutkowska K, Oprządek J, et al. Genetic disorders in beef cattle: a review. Genes Genomics 2017;39(5):461–71.

18. Cole JB. A simple strategy for managing many recessive disorders in a dairy cattle breeding program. Genet Sel Evol 2015;47(1). https://doi.org/10.1186/s12711-015-0174-9.

19. Kemper KE, Goddard ME. Understanding and predicting complex traits: knowledge from cattle. Hum Mol Genet 2012;21(R1):R45–51.

20. Daetwyler HD, Capitan A, Pausch H, et al. Whole-genome sequencing of 234 bulls facilitates mapping of monogenic and complex traits in cattle. Nat Genet 2014;46(8):858–65.

21. Xiang R, van den Berg I, MacLeod IM, et al. Quantifying the contribution of sequence variants with regulatory and evolutionary significance to 34 bovine complex traits. Proc Natl Acad Sci U S A 2019;116(39):19398–408.

22. Hill WG, Mackay TFCDS. Falconer and Introduction to quantitative genetics. Genetics 2004;167(4):1529–36.

23. Hill WG, Goddard ME, Visscher PM. Data and theory point to mainly additive genetic variance for complex traits. PLoS Genet 2008;4(2):e1000008.

24. Fisher RA. XV.—The Correlation between Relatives on the Supposition of Mendelian Inheritance. Earth Environ Sci Trans R Soc Edinb 1919;52(2):399–433.

25. Abdollahi-Arpanahi R, Lourenco D, Legarra A, et al. Dissecting genetic trends to understand breeding practices in livestock: a maternal pig line example. Genet Sel Evol 2021;53(1):89.

26. Lush JL. Animal breeding plans. Ames, IA: Iowa State College Press; 1965.

27. Hill WG. Understanding and using quantitative genetic variation. Philos Trans R Soc Lond B Biol Sci 2010;365(1537):73–85.

28. Land RB, Hill WG. The possible use of superovulation and embryo transfer in cattle to increase response to selection. Anim Sci 1975;21(1):1–12.

29. Koch RM, Gregory KE, Cundiff LV. Selection in Beef Cattle II. Selection Response2. J Anim Sci 1974;39(3):459–70.

30. Morrissey MB, Kruuk LEB, Wilson AJ. The danger of applying the breeder's equation in observational studies of natural populations. J Evol Biol 2010;23(11):2277–88.

31. García-Ruiz A, Cole JB, VanRaden PM, et al. Changes in genetic selection differentials and generation intervals in US Holstein dairy cattle as a result of genomic selection. Proc. Natl. Acad. Sci. U.S.A 2016;113(28):E3995–4004.

32. Hazel LN. The Genetic Basis for Constructing Selection Indexes. Genetics 1943; 28(6):476–90.

33. Henderson CR. Best linear unbiased estimation and prediction under a selection model. Biometrics 1975;31(2):423–47.

34. Meuwissen TH, Hayes BJ, Goddard ME. Prediction of total genetic value using genome-wide dense marker maps. Genetics 2001;157(4):1819–29.

35. Bourdon RM. Understanding Animal Breeding, 2. Essex, England: Pearson Education; 2014.

36. Meuwissen T, Hayes B, Goddard M. Accelerating improvement of livestock with genomic selection. Annu Rev Anim Biosci 2013;1(1):221–37.

37. Loi P, Toschi P, Zacchini F, et al. Synergies between assisted reproduction technologies and functional genomics. Genet Sel Evol 2016;48(1):53.

38. Gonzalez-Recio O, Coffey MP, Pryce JE. On the value of the phenotypes in the genomic era. J Dairy Sci 2014;97(12):7905–15.

39. Daetwyler HD, Villanueva B, Woolliams JA. Accuracy of predicting the genetic risk of disease using a genome-wide approach. PLoS One 2008;3(10):e3395.

40. Sorensen DA, Kennedy BW. Estimation of response to selection using least-squares and mixed model methodology. J Anim Sci 1984;58(5):1097–106.

41. van Bebber J, Reinsch N, Junge W, et al. Accounting for herd, year and season effects in genetic evaluations of dairy cattle: a review. Livest Prod Sci 1997; 51(1–3):191–203.

42. Van Vleck LD. Contemporary groups for genetic evaluations. J Dairy Sci 1987; 70(11):2456–64.

43. Garrick DJ. The nature, scope and impact of genomic prediction in beef cattle in the United States. Genet Sel Evol 2011;43(1):17.

44. McHugh N, Pabiou T, Wall E, et al. Impact of alternative definitions of contemporary groups on genetic evaluations of traits recorded at lambing1. J Anim Sci 2017;95(5):1926–38.

45. Gorjanc G, Bijma P, Hickey JM. Reliability of pedigree-based and genomic evaluations in selected populations. Genet Sel Evol 2015;47(1). https://doi.org/10.1186/s12711-015-0145-1.

46. Wright S. Systems of mating. I. The biometric relations between parent and offspring. Genetics 1921;6(2):111–23.

47. Van Vleck LD. Computing numerator relationships between any pair of animals. Genet Mol Res 2007;6(3):685–90.

48. Pimentel ECG, Edel C, Emmerling R, et al. How pedigree errors affect genetic evaluations and validation statistics. J Dairy Sci 2023. https://doi.org/10.3168/jds.2023-24070.

49. US Council on Dairy Cattle Breeding. CBCD Services. Available at: https://uscdcb.com/services/. [Accessed 27 March 2024].

50. International Genetic Solutions. Multi-breed evaluation. Available at: https://www.internationalgeneticsolutions.com/site/index.php/multi-breed-genetic-evaluation. [Accessed 27 March 2024].

51. Schaeffer LR. Animal models. Volumes direct; 2019.

52. Rowan TN. Invited Review: Genetic decision tools for increasing cow efficiency and sustainability in forage-based beef systems. Applied Animal Science 2022; 38(6):660–70.

53. Oliveira Junior GA, Schenkel FS, Alcantara L, et al. Estimated genetic parameters for all genetically evaluated traits in Canadian Holsteins. J Dairy Sci 2021;104(8): 9002–15.
54. Wiggans GR, Carrillo JA. Genomic selection in United States dairy cattle. Front Genet 2022;13. https://doi.org/10.3389/fgene.2022.994466.
55. Seidel A, Krattenmacher N, Thaller G. Dealing with complexity of new phenotypes in modern dairy cattle breeding. Anim Front 2020;10(2):23–8.
56. Hayes BJ, Bowman PJ, Chamberlain AJ, et al. Invited review: Genomic selection in dairy cattle: progress and challenges. J Dairy Sci 2009;92(2):433–43.
57. Slatkin M. Linkage disequilibrium–understanding the evolutionary past and mapping the medical future. Nat Rev Genet 2008;9(6):477–85.
58. VanRaden PM. Efficient methods to compute genomic predictions. J Dairy Sci 2008;91(11):4414–23.
59. Robertson A, Rendel JM. The use of progeny testing with artificial insemination in dairy cattle. J Genet 1950;50(1):21–31.
60. Matukumalli LK, Lawley CT, Schnabel RD, et al. Development and characterization of a high density SNP genotyping assay for cattle. PLoS One 2009;4(4):e5350.
61. Rolf MM, Taylor JF, Schnabel RD, et al. Impact of reduced marker set estimation of genomic relationship matrices on genomic selection for feed efficiency in Angus cattle. BMC Genet 2010;11:24.
62. MacLeod IM, Bowman PJ, Vander Jagt CJ, et al. Exploiting biological priors and sequence variants enhances QTL discovery and genomic prediction of complex traits. BMC Genom 2016;17:144.
63. Snelling WM, Hoff JL, Li JH, et al. Assessment of Imputation from Low-Pass Sequencing to Predict Merit of Beef Steers. Genes 2020;11(11). https://doi.org/10.3390/genes11111312.
64. Li JH, Mazur CA, Berisa T, et al. Low-pass sequencing increases the power of GWAS and decreases measurement error of polygenic risk scores compared to genotyping arrays. Genome Res 2021;31(4):529–37.

Beef Genetic Evaluations

Matthew L. Spangler, PhD, MS (Animal Breeding and Genetics), BS (Anim Sciences)[a],*, Donagh P. Berry, PhD, MSc Bioinformatics, BSc[b]

KEYWORDS

- Cattle • Estimated breeding value • Expected progeny difference • Genomics
- Economic selection index

KEY POINTS

- Routine genetic evaluations rely on known kinship among animals, accurately-recorded phenotypic records, and known and accurately-recorded systematic effects.
- Genomic data have led to increased accuracy of resulting genetic predictions particularly at younger ages, offering the potential for faster rates of annual genetic gain.
- Economic selection indexes enable selection for multiple traits simultaneously in an economic framework, even if antagonistically correlated.
- Using genetic predictions and economic selection indexes requires identification of and adherence to a well-defined breeding objective.

INTRODUCTION

Formal genetic evaluations of beef cattle, akin to what is in existence today, have been in existence for over 50 years.[1] Underlying the system of genetic evaluation is the fact that observable and quantifiable characteristics of animals are heritable. Consequently, selection of parental animals based on heritable traits can lead to changes in the population. However, not all variation among animals is due to variation in genetics, with management and production environments playing a non-negligible role that varies in proportionality by trait. The role of genetic evaluations, therefore, is to disentangle such genetic and non-genetic effects, and in doing so, generate estimates of genetic merit that are independent of non-genetic effects. These estimates are called Estimated Breeding Values (EBV) although some countries (ie, the United States [US]) provide industry with Expected Progeny Differences (EPD), which are simply half of an EBV; some countries like Ireland present these as Predicted Transmitting Ability estimates that are akin to EPD, but is the terminology commonly used in dairy cattle breeding.

Understandably, the first traits evaluated were those that were easiest to collect; thus, the first genetic predictions in many countries were for birth, weaning (direct

a Department of Animal Science, University of Nebraska-Lincoln, Lincoln, NE, USA; b Animal & Grassland Research and Innovation Centre, Teagasc, Moorepark, Fermoy, Cork, Ireland
* Corresponding author.
E-mail address: mspangler2@unl.edu

Vet Clin Food Anim 40 (2024) 357–367
https://doi.org/10.1016/j.cvfa.2024.05.002   vetfood.theclinics.com
0749-0720/24/© 2024 Elsevier Inc. All rights reserved, including that for text and data mining, AI training, and similar technologies.

and maternal), and yearling weight.[1] Over time, the list of traits evaluated has expanded considerably and now includes female fertility, carcass merit, feed intake, and traits related to management and animal well-being, such as temperament, teat and udder scores, and feet and leg conformation. As contemplation of the impact of animals on their environment gains more attention, genetic predictions for environmental footprint traits, such as methane output or intensity, have also been investigated.[2] As the list of traits with available genetic predictions increases, the actual selection decision-making process by producers becomes arguably more complicated; a classical *information overload* problem. The derivation of breeding objectives,[3] or goals, and selection based on economic selection indexes[4] that align with the identified objective becomes key not only to reduce complexity, but also to ensure selection decisions lead to cumulative and sustainable improvements in net profit.

In addition to generating predictions for more traits, considerable emphasis has been placed on improving the accuracy of these genetic predictions. The statistical framework for modern genetic evaluations is the Mixed Model Equations (MME).[5,6] Although the general framework has remained the same for decades, substantive changes have been made to better utilize the data available and thus produce estimates that are more accurate. The implementation of advanced statistical models has often been accompanied by advances in computational software and hardware, enabling timely delivery of genetic predictions to the end users. Most recently, genomic data have been integrated into prediction models,[7–9] leading to increased accuracy of genetic predictions most notably for young animals.

Despite the substantial advances in genetic evaluations, and the evidence that these predictions indeed work,[10] adoption of available genetic selection tools by industry is less than desirable, at least in some countries.[11,12] The reasons for low adoption rates are likely many including the before mentioned information overload problem, uncertainty relative to how such predictions are derived, simple traditional precedent, and fundamental lack of understanding of the interpretation of the predictions themselves perhaps leading to incorrect expectations. In some countries, there still exists a tradition of placing considerable emphasis on the observable features of natural mating bulls when making a purchasing decision.

The focus herein is on the history of beef cattle genetic evaluations, their current purpose and state, and their likely future. The principle emphasis is a high-level description of how genetic evaluations work and the use of resulting genetic predictions in delivering sustainable genetic gain.

Purpose and Historical Context

The notion of performance recording in cattle is thought to date back to Roman times.[13] Robert Bakewell (1725–1795) is often acknowledged as one of the first to implement systematic breeding and is often dubbed the father of modern animal breeding. Bakewell's ability to *"modify [...] the forms and qualities of [...] cattle"* was actually recognized in Darwin's "On the Origin of Species by Means of Natural Selection".[14] However, it was not until the establishment of breed societies and herdbooks around the 1800s[15] that performance recording began in cattle began. In the US, 5 beef breed associations had initiated performance recording programs by 1964.[1] Prior to the advent of these recording programs, and arguably still after, selection criteria were based on visual assessment.[1] The notion of being able to visually assess the genetic potential of an animal for an array of quantitative traits that describe an economically-driven breeding objective, as well as partition the differences observed between that which is heritable and that which is non-genetic is an impossible task.

Accurate performance records have a multitude of uses including benchmarking herd performance against contemporaries, monitoring of temporal trends in herd performance (ie, evaluation of changes in management practices such as diet), monitoring individual animals temporally for changes in performance as an indicator of some underlying issues, benchmarking animals within herd to aid culling, and genetic evaluations. The purpose of genetic evaluations is to quantify the differences among candidate parents for traits that are deemed important to industry and by doing so, enabling incremental changes in the performance metrics of commercial animals. Modern genetic evaluations are strongly underpinned by statistical methods that enable the disentanglement of genetic and non-genetic sources of variation to ultimately generate EBV, which are the estimates of genetic merit of individual animals, each with an associated accuracy or reliability.

Current genetic evaluations use a set of statistical models called the MME first proposed by Henderson.[5,6] In matrix notation, the model equation for a simple univariate analysis with no repeated records could be represented as follows:

$$y = Xb + Zu + e$$

where y represents a vector of observations for the trait of interest (eg, weight, carcass trait, and fertility observation), b represents a vector of fixed effects (eg, non-genetic sources of variation such as sex, age), u represents a vector of random additive genetic effects (breeding values), e represents a vector of random residual components, which is part of the phenotype not explained by effects in b or u. The X and Z matrices relate observations in y to fixed effects in b and random additive genetic effects in u, respectively. The adoption of the MME that provide Best Linear Unbiased Predictions (BLUP) of breeding values enabled all the data to be used by improving predictions across contemporary groups (ie, herd-year combinations).[5] Comparisons across time and across herds was also aided by advancements in reproductive technology and the adoption of artificial insemination, which facilitated common sires and ancestors across herds.

Traits which were initially the focus of genetic evaluations were those that were easiest to quantify, such as weight. Consequently, early EPD in the US were for early growth traits such as weight at birth, weaning, and yearling. As both statistical models and the ability to collect phenotypes matured, the depth and breadth of traits explored for genetic predictions expanded (**Table 1**).

Genetic Evaluation Process

Genetic evaluations are enabled by the data sharing among participating breeders. The conduit for sharing is the genetic evaluation or the database(s) that contribute to it. Breeders often submit the data to an organization (eg, breed association, national, or centralized repository) and that entity then submit the data to the genetic evaluation, or indeed itself undertakes the genetic evaluation. The entity that conducts genetic evaluations can take on 3 general forms: a breed association or society, a governmental agency, or a private firm. In some cases multiple entities, like individual breed associations, may collaborate and conduct a joint genetic evaluation that includes the data from multiple breed associations. Some breeders may also participate in multiple genetic evaluations by recording animals with more than 1 breed association. The entire infrastructure is greatly simplified in countries where a single entity conducts a unified genetic evaluation across all herds as exists in Ireland. The data submitted must adhere to specified definitions dictated by the genetic evaluation provider in terms of age ranges when weights can be collected, and animal identification conventions.

Table 1
Traits with estimated breeding values (EBV) published in either the U.S. or Ireland

Trait	US	Ireland
Growth		
Direct/maternal birth weight	X	
Direct/maternal Weaning weight	X	X
Yearling/400d weight	X	
ADG	X	
Mature or cull cow weight	X	X
Mature height	X	
Yearling height	X	
Carcass		
Weight	X	X
Conformation		X
Subcutaneous fat cover/depth	X	X
Ultrasound Eye muscle area	X	
Warner-Bratzler shear force	X	
Carcass eye muscle area	X	
Intramuscular fat/marbling	X	
Yield grade	X	
Linear classification		
Skeletal at weaning		X
Muscle at weaning		X
Functional at weaning		X
Feed intake complex		
Feed intake	X	X
Feed efficiency	X	
Ultrasound		
Fat	X	
Rib eye area	X	
Intermuscular fat	X	
Reproduction		
Days to calving	X	
Calving interval		X
Pregnancy/non-return rate	X	
Survival/longevity/stayability	X	X
Scrotal circumference	X	
Age at first calving	X	X
Health		
TB		X
Liver fluke		X
Hair shedding	X	
Pulmonary arterial pressure	X	
Calving performance		
Direct calving difficulty	X	X

(continued on next page)

Table 1 (continued)		
Trait	**US**	**Ireland**
Maternal calving difficulty	X	X
Direct gestation length		X
Maternal gestation length		
Direct stillbirth		X
Welfare		
Body condition score	X	X
Udder traits	X	
Feet & legs traits	X	
Environmental traits		
Methane emissions		X
Management		
Docility	X	X

List of traits is current as of February 2024. The listing of traits in the US varies by breed association.

The data submitted to a genetic evaluation are often subjected to quality control procedures, which can be as simple as rules-based approaches that discard the data above or below certain thresholds or based on extremeness determined by the extent of deviations from a mean value. More sophisticated approaches that employ deep learning models have also been used to aid in categorizing the data based on quality.[16] The other quality control component is pedigree integrity, which has been greatly enhanced using genomics. Genomic data can validate that the proposed parents are indeed the parents of a given offspring. Genomic information can also be used to discover the true parent(s) of an offspring and in fact, can actually circumvent the necessity for recording ancestry information through the construction of relationships via the extent of DNA shared among animals.

Once the genetic evaluation is completed, additional checks are often performed to ensure the resulting outputs (ie, EBV and associated accuracy metrics) are reliable and often include a comparison of EBV from the current evaluation to the previous evaluation to determine if ranking, particularly among high accuracy sires, is relatively stable. Genetic evaluations in beef cattle in the US were historically conducted twice annually to coincide with 2 calving seasons (spring and fall), while other countries such as Ireland conducted evaluations 4 times per year. However, the widespread use of genotyping with medium-density single nucleotide polymorphism arrays led to more frequent genetic evaluations in those countries that historically had less frequent evaluations. Understandably, if producers made an investment in genotyping they wanted to see the resulting change in EBV sooner than in several months' time. Currently, genetic evaluations are conducted weekly in the US.

Traits

The list of traits has expanded due to changes in the ability to collect phenotypes (eg, carcass ultrasound), advancements in the statistical models used to accommodate serially recorded traits like reproductive success across parities using random regression,[17] and changes in the economic signals received by industry, necessitating focus on additional traits (eg, methane emissions).

Table 1 contains a listing of traits currently evaluated in the US and Ireland. Although there are similarities between them, obvious differences exist. These differences can be attributed to 2 primary factors: industry structure and economic drivers of the commercial industry. In the US, genetic evaluations are (largely) either conducted by or coordinated by beef breed associations and rely predominantly on the data derived from the seed stock sector. In contrast, Ireland benefits from a single centralized national database and associated genetic evaluation platform that is powered primarily by the data from the commercial sector, at least in part enabled by a mandatory national animal identification program, and associated tracking system and exchequer support for data recording.

It is highly likely that additional traits will be added to evaluations in the future. Traits related to disease such as bovine respiratory disease complex, male fertility, additional traits related to female fertility, and characteristics of beef that drive consumer satisfaction and demand are all possibilities assuming data collection schemes can be justified to enable genetic evaluation for these traits. There is also mounting evidence that suggests features of the rumen microbiome are heritable,[18] yet taking this knowledge to the point of genetic evaluation requires considerable research effort.

Genomics

Genomic technology initially served as a disrupter to traditional genetic evaluations in beef cattle. Commercial companies marketed tests that delivered scores (eg, 1–10, number of stars) to producers from which to rank animals based on genetic potential from the genomic test. Simultaneously, seed stock animals were also evaluated by national or international genetic evaluations that generated EBV. These 2 values per animal (ie, EBV and the results from the genomic test) were then used by producers to make decisions. This was an unworkable task, given there is no clear way to use these 2 disjoined, yet dependent, metrics to make coherent selection decisions. This was exacerbated by the fact that these commercialized genomic tests were shown to have low accuracy in some populations.[19] Ultimately genetic evaluations began using the results from genomic tests as a supplementary source of information in the genetic prediction procedures through either blending of pedigree-based EBV and genomic predictors' post genetic evaluation, or using multi-trait model approaches.[20,21] Currently, genomic data are, in many countries, incorporated into genetic evaluations using 'single-step' models that directly fit the genotypes, rather than a prediction based from them, into the genetic evaluation.[7–9] The 2 primary methods currently used to incorporate the genomic data into routine genetic evaluations in several populations are single-step genomic BLUP[7] and single step Bayesian regression.[9] These 2 modeling approaches are equivalent given certain circumstances.[9] The use of the genomic data does differ by evaluation; some genomic evaluations may elect to place more or less emphasis on the genomic information relative to that captured by the ancestral information. Regardless of the nuances of the statistical models used, the inclusion of the genomic data has proven beneficial in improving the accuracy of EBV, particularly for young animals. This increase in accuracy for young animals is driven by improved estimates of relationships among animals beyond the expected, or average, values assumed by pedigree. In many US breeds that have adopted the use of genomic prediction, the value of genotyping non-parent animals has been illustrated by calculating progeny equivalents. These progeny equivalent values represent the number of phenotyped and recorded offspring that an animal would need to have produced in order to achieve the same level of accuracy as the genomic data alone would provide. Depending on trait and breed, these values can range from approximately 5 to 25, meaning that genotyping a non-parent bull can provide the same level of accuracy as if he had already sired 5 to 25 offspring.

Genomic selection in beef cattle is relatively new. Rostam and colleagues used the historic data in 3 species to estimate the initiation of genomic selection in each species using differences between genetic trends and trends in realized mendelian sampling.[22] Mendelian sampling is the random assortment of alleles from parent to offspring, and is perhaps most tangibly thought of as the genetic variation among full siblings. In a random mating population, the realized Mendelian sampling is expected to be 0 given no artificial selection is being practiced and the mean genetic value of parents is expected to be the same as the offspring. In populations undergoing selection the realized Mendelian sampling will not be 0, but should be close to it.[22] In American Angus cattle, trends for realized Mendelian sampling only began diverging from genetic trends in 2009 for weaning weight and 2016 for postweaning gain,[22] suggesting that the full impacts of genomic selection have yet to be observed. Moreover, Rostam and colleagues noted the presence of selective genotyping whereby decisions of which animals to genotype were conditional on phenotypic performance for early growth traits (eg, weaning weight).[22] Ideally, all animals would be genotyped and any culling decisions made based on genomic EBV. Moreover, genomic data by itself are of no value for predicting genetic merit from complex traits. Consequently, organizations need to minimally maintain and ideally bolster phenotypic recording schemes to better leverage the benefit of genomic prediction. This is particularly true for sex-limited traits such as female fertility, traits that can only be recorded on harvested animals such as carcass records, traits related to disease, and traits of emerging societal importance (eg, methane emissions).

Use and Interpretation of Genetic Predictions

Predictions from genetic evaluations are generally reported in units of the trait (if such exists), with some exceptions where the EBV or EPD are reported on a probabilistic scale (ie, more likely to produce offspring that are docile or more likely to produce offspring that are born unassisted). Entities that conduct genetic evaluations frequently publish summary statistics, such as the mean (breed average) and percentile ranks to help guide users in determining the relative ranking of individuals for each trait evaluated. Additionally, accuracy values reflect the degree to which an animal's prediction could change with additional information. Accuracy itself can be confusing given its many definitions. Although the range is bounded by 0 and 1, different countries report different metrics associated with accuracy. Theoretically, accuracy is the correlation between the prediction (EBV) and true genetic merit of an individual, but is approximated[23] and the model derived values are reported as part of the deliverables to producers. Some entities report the square of accuracy, called reliability. Yet other entities, like the US, report accuracy on the Beef Improvement Federation scale that is much more conservative.[24] In all cases, the value of accuracy is often misinterpreted by practitioners. A much more intuitive measure to report alongside the estimate of genetic merit would be a confidence interval that can be generated with knowledge of the EBV or EPD and the standard error of prediction. Most beef breed associations in the US do publish a possible change table that can be used to construct confidence intervals, although directly supplying this value would be ideal. For those that might use multiple sires, as could be the case in extensive production systems where breeding pastures could include several natural service sires, the accuracy of the average EBV of the bulls is the most important metric and the accuracy of this average is considerably greater than the accuracy of any individual bull contained in the group.

Unfortunately, EBV or EPD is not always directly comparable across country or even within country or across breeds. These incompatibilities arise for 3 general reasons: different base adjustment, a lack of connectivity (eg, genetic links), and 2 (or more) evaluations within breed in the same country but performed by different entities. A base relative to EPD or EBV is often set as a point in time or a set of reference animals for which all other EBV or EPD are relative to. This differs among genetic evaluations. The lack of genetic connectivity arises due to a lack of kinship ties. A singular genetic evaluation within a country solves the base issue and if a there are crossbred records that enter an evaluation, then connectivity can exist across breeds. In the US, the EPD from several breed associations are not directly comparable and across-breed adjustment factors published annually by the US Meat Animal Research Center are needed to place animals on a common base to directly compare EPD.[10] In countries like Ireland, all animals of all breeds (including dairy) are evaluated in a common evaluation (for some traits) thereby enabling a direct comparison of animals of all breeds (and crossbreds) on the same scale; this is enabled by a centralized database and national genetic evaluation system underpinning by the predominantly crossbred data. Because, crossbred beef cattle predominate in Ireland, the industry demands an across-breed genetic evaluation system.

Breeding Objectives

Estimates of genetic merit, EBV or EPD, can be used to directionally change populations. However, if the goal is to improve the profitability and more broadly the sustainability of individual enterprises and an entire industry, then selection must contemplate intermediate levels of performance as opposed to a mantra of continually increasing or decreasing a particular trait. To select for improved sustainability (including economic, environmental, and societal sustainability) then a breeding objective must first be defined in such a way that these 3 areas are explicitly defined, and therefore economic costs or returns can be assigned to them. At a high level, a breeding objective should define the point of sale for terminal calves (eg, at weaning, after a backgrounding period, after the finishing phase, etc.), if female replacements will be retained or not, and environmental or labor constraints. These broad characterizations of the objectives of an enterprise help define the traits that are economically relevant to the enterprise. For example, if a producer retains all animals (males and females) through the finishing phase and markets them toward a program that rewards high-yielding and high-marbling carcasses, then the breeding objective is defined by traits of terminal importance such as feed intake, carcass weight, carcass marbling, components of carcass yield, and susceptibility to disease. However, if the goal includes the retention of replacement females, then the list of traits that impact net profit would expand to include traits related to female fertility or longevity, cow cost (eg, mature cow weight), maternal calving ease, and so forth. Once a breeding objective is identified, a phenotypic data collection scheme conditioned on the breeding objective to ensure the data for objective traits, or at least those reasonably genetically correlated with them, should be in order. This is in stark contrast to building an objective around a list of existing traits for which genetic predictions are made.

Breeding objectives inherently are comprised of more than 1 trait and thus, selection for multiple traits simultaneously is required to make progress in the breeding objective. Selection index theory represents a means of weighting each trait differently to form an index to use as the selection criterion.[25,26] An economic selection index should align with the identified breeding objective, such that selection on and eventual increases in index values of animals should translate into progress in the breeding objective and thus, improvements in net profit for commercial herds. The traits in the index do not need to match one-to-one the traits in the breeding objective, but estimates of the genetic relationships between the objective traits and the index traits should be estimated.[27] Identifying a breeding objective and corresponding economic selection index are not trivial exercises. In addition to identifying traits that are economically relevant,[28] a breeding objective and associated index needs to contemplate the planning horizon that the commercial producer desires to determine the costs and returns associated with a selection decision. The planning horizon impacts the number of discounted expressions of a given trait.[29,30] Valasek and colleagues illustrated that, for a general-purpose index where replacement females were retained and all male offspring and cull heifers were sold at weaning, the relative emphasis of stability (sustained cow fertility) was near 0% at very short (ie, 2-year) planning horizons, but greater than 30% once the planning horizon extended beyond 20 years.[30] This is a function of the number of expressions of sustained cow fertility that can be observed in 2 years versus 20 years; traits expressed later in life increase in relative importance as the length of the planning horizon increases. Moreover, current levels of herd or population performance can impact the weighting of traits in an index. As phenotypic levels of performance approach pricing thresholds (discounts or premiums), the marginal economic value associated with the trait changes.[30] Consequently, entities need to re-evaluate the economic weights used in indexes accordingly as populations change.

Although genetic evaluations produce useful information from which to help make decisions (EBV), considerable work is required to bridge the gap between enterprise level objectives, an expanding list of EBV, and selection decisions. The notion of decision support is not new,[31] but availability and adoption of such tools in beef cattle breeding can be bolstered. Currently, examples do exist such as iGENDEC[32] in the US and BreedObject in Australia,[33] but effort will no doubt be required to maintain and expand the utility and application of such tools to enhance decision support.

SUMMARY

Genetic evaluations have continually evolved as advancements in statistical methods, computational improvements, the available data, and industry needs have emerged. The results of routine genetic evaluations, EBV, are a stark improvement compared to any other method of ranking selection candidates. The use of genomic information as an added data source in genetic evaluations has increased the accuracy of EBV and offered the opportunity to accelerate genetic change. To fully exploit the utility of genomic data, all animals must be genotyped and decisions taken using the EBV enhanced with genomic data. Progress, however, must be conditioned on a pertinent breeding objective and selection decisions taken based on an economic selection index that is aligned with the breeding objective(s) identified. As the list of traits evaluated continues to grow, care should be given as to what is actually published and provided to cattle breeding practitioners to avoid an overwhelming amount of different information, many of which can be antagonistically correlated.

CLINICS CARE POINTS

- Genetic predictions (EBV or EPD), like all predictions, are associated with some degree of error or uncertainty. The confidence in genetic predictions is quantified by the associated accuracy or reliability.
- Genetically superior parents can produce poor performing offspring due to Mendelian sampling and the environmental or management effects on the trait.

- Genetic evaluations are conditional on the data provided. All else being equal, more accurate data, kinship and phenotypes, leads to more accurate predictions
- Genomic data increase the accuracy of resulting genetic predictions but require that there be continual collection of phenotypes.
- Generating a breeding objective and making genetic selection decisions based on the breeding objective using economic selection indexes, simplifies selection decisions and leads to improved net profit.
- EBV or EPD are tools for making comparisons among animals, and knowledge of population (breed) averages is important. Not all EBV or EPD are directly comparable across countries or even within country and across breeds.

DISCLOSURE

The authors have no conflict of interest.

REFERENCES

1. Golden BL, Garrick DJ, Benyshek LL. Milestones in beef cattle genetic evaluation. J Anim Sci 2009;87(ESuppl):E3–10.
2. Donoghue KA, Bird-Gardiner T, Arthur PF, et al. Genetic and phenotypic variance and covariance components for methane emission and postweaning traits in angus cattle. J Anim Sci 2016;94:1438–45.
3. Goddard ME. Consensus and debate in the definition of breeding objectives. J Dairy Sci 1998;81:6–18.
4. MacNeil MD, Newman S, Enns RM, et al. Relative economic values for Canadian beef production using specialized sire and dam lines. Can J Anim Sci 1994;74:411–7.
5. Henderson CR. Best linear unbiased estimation and prediction under a selection model. Biometrics 1975;31:423–47.
6. Henderson CR. In: Shaeffer LR, editor. Applications of linear models in animal breeding. Guelph: University of Guelph; 1984.
7. Legarra A, Aguilar I, Misztal I. A relationship matrix including full pedigree and genomic information. J Dairy Sci 2009;92:4656–63.
8. Christensen OF, Lund MS. Genomic prediction when some animals are not genotyped. Genet Sel Evol 2010;42:2–10.
9. Fernando RL, Dekkers JC, Garrick DJ. A class of Bayesian methods to combine large numbers of genotyped and non-genotyped animals for whole-genome analyses. Genet Sel Evol 2014;46:50.
10. Kuehn LA, Thallman RM. Across-breed EPD tables for the year 2017 adjusted to breed differences for birth year of 2015. Proc. Beef Imp. Fed., 48th Ann. Res. Symp. & Ann. Meet 2017;112–44.
11. Weaber RL, Beever JE, Freetly HC, et al. Analysis of US Cow-Calf Producer Survey Data to Assess Knowledge, Awareness and Attitudes Related to Genetic Improvement of Feed Efficiency. In: Proc. 10th world congress on genetics applied to livestock production. 2014.
12. Weaber RL, Kuehn LA, Snelling WM, et al. Beef Cattle Genetic Technology Utilization - Survey of Stakeholders. J Anim Sci 2019;97(Suppl. 3).
13. Turner H. Coat characters of cattle in relation to adaptation. In: Proceedings of the Australian society of animal production. 1964.
14. Darwin C. On the Origin of species by means of natural selection, or preservation of favoured races in the struggle for life. London: John Murray; 1859.

15. Brotherstone S, Goddard M. Artificial selection and maintenance of genetic variance in the global dairy cow population. Philos Trans R Soc Lond B Biol 2005; 360:1479–88.
16. Ribeiro A, Golden BL, Spangler ML. Categorization of birth weight phenotypes for inclusion in genetic evaluations using a Deep Neural Network. J Anim Sci 2021; 99:skab053.
17. Jamrozik JS, McGrath S, Kemp RA, et al. Estimates of genetic parameters for stayability to consecutive calvings of Canadian Simmentals by random regression models. J Anim Sci 2013;91:3634–43.
18. Waseem A, Howard JT, Paz HA, et al. Influence of host genetics in shaping the rumen bacterial community in beef cattle. Sci Rep 2020;10:15101.
19. Van Eenennaam AL, Li J, Thallman RM, et al. Validation of commercial DNA tests for quantitative beef quality traits. J Anim Sci 2007;85:891–900.
20. Kachman S. Incorporation of marker scores into national cattle evaluations. Kansas City, MO: Proc. 9th Genetic Prediction Workshop; 2008. p. 88–91.
21. MacNeil MD, Nkrumah JD, Woodward BW, et al. Genetic evaluation of Angus cattle for carcass marbling using ultrasound and genomic indicators. J Anim Sci 2010;88:517–30.
22. Rostam AA, Lourenco D, Misztal I. Detecting effective starting point of genomic selection by divergent trends from best linear unbiased prediction and single-step genomic best linear unbiased prediction in pigs, beef cattle, and broilers. J Anim Sci 2021;99:1–11.
23. Harris B, Johnson D. Approximate reliability of genetic evaluations under an animal model. J Dairy Sci 1988;10:2723–8.
24. Improvement Federation Beef. Guidelines for uniform beef improvement programs. Available at: https://guidelines.beefimprovement.org/index.php/Accuracy. [Accessed 1 February 2024].
25. Hazel LN, Lush JL. The efficiency of three methods of selection. J Hered 1942;33:393–9.
26. Hazel LN. The genetic basis for constructing selection indexes. Genetics 1943;28:476–90.
27. Ochsner KP, MacNeil MD, Lewis RM, et al. Economic selection index development for Beefmaster cattle II: General-purpose breeding objective. J Anim Sci 2017;95:1913–20.
28. Golden BL, Garrick DJ, Newman S, et al. A framework for the next generation of EPD. Proc. Beef Improv. Fed. 32nd Ann. Res. Symp. Annu. Meet 2000;32:2–13.
29. Amer PR. Economic accounting of numbers of expressions and delays in sheep genetic improvement. N Z J Agric Res 1999;42:325–36.
30. Valasek H.F., Golden B.L., Spangler M.L., Impact of planning horizon length on the relative emphasis of traits in economic breeding goals. Proc. 12th World Congress on Genetics Applied to Livestock Production, July 3-8, 2022. Rotterdam, The Netherlands, 2022.
31. Newman S, Lynch T, Plummer AA. Success and failure of decision support systems: Learning as we go. J Anim Sci 2000;77:1–12.
32. Spangler M.L., Golden B.L., Newman S., et al., iGENDEC: a web-based decision support tool for economic index construction. Proc. 12th World Congress on Genetics Applied to Livestock Production, July 3-8, 2022. Rotterdam, The Netherlands, 2022.
33. Barwick SA, Henzell AL. Development successes and issues for the future in deriving and applying selection indexes for beef breeding. Aust J Exp Agric 2005;45:923–33.

Innovating Beef Cattle Veterinary Practices
Leveraging Genetic and Genomic Tools

Maci L. Mueller, PhD[a],*, Jamie T. Courter, PhD[b], Randall Spare, DVM[c]

KEYWORDS

- Beef cattle • Bovine • Veterinarian • Genetic selection • Genomic selection
- Calving ease

KEY POINTS

- Beef cattle veterinarians, as trusted sources of information, now serve as proactive advisors beyond disease treatment.
- Beef cattle veterinarians with knowledge of genetic tools are poised to be vital in addressing modern beef industry challenges.
- Genetic selection for calving ease traits is a key strategy to minimize dystocia, highlighting the role of a genetic approach in enhancing animal health and welfare.
- Both seedstock and commercial producers now have access to a range of genomic technologies, with investment levels directly determining the extent of genomic insights gained.
- Integrating genomic data with veterinary insights, such as pregnancy and fetal sex information, allow for each animal to be directed through a specific value-added market to optimize economic returns.

INTRODUCTION

Veterinarians have long been and remain a cornerstone of support for beef cattle producers, offering expert guidance on a wide array of topics including animal health, nutrition, and production management.[1,2] This enduring relationship underscores the critical role that veterinarians fulfill within the beef cattle industry. While traditionally focusing on disease treatment, the function of beef cattle veterinarians has broadened significantly to include disease prevention and the enhancement of productivity and economic resilience in beef production.

[a] Department of Animal Sciences and Industry, Kansas State University, 1424 Claflin Road, 242 Weber Hall, Manhattan, KS 66506, USA; [b] Division of Animal Sciences, University of Missouri, 920 East Campus Drive, Columbia, MO 65211, USA; [c] Ashland Veterinary Center Inc., P.O. Box 869, West Highway 160, Ashland, KS 67831, USA
* Corresponding author. Department of Animal Sciences and Industry, Kansas State University, 1424 Claflin Road, 242 Weber Hall, Manhattan, KS 66506.
E-mail address: muellermaci@ksu.edu
Twitter: @maci_mueller (M.L.M.)

Vet Clin Food Anim 40 (2024) 369–380
https://doi.org/10.1016/j.cvfa.2024.05.004
0749-0720/24/Published by Elsevier Inc.

vetfood.theclinics.com

To effectively meet the challenges posed by both traditional responsibilities and the demands of modern beef production, bovine veterinarians must embrace innovative tools and technologies. Notably, an understanding of genetics and selection tools available enables veterinarians to ask the right questions and address the fundamental challenges impacting animal health, welfare, and production efficiency.

This article will first illustrate a key example of how genetic selection can directly promote animal health and welfare, specifically focusing on addressing calving difficulties. Additionally, the opportunity to integrate genomic data with veterinary expertise to enable both seedstock and commercial producers to execute informed decisions regarding selection, mating, and marketing strategies will be discussed. By delving into these topics, this article aims to showcase the critical importance of a progressive approach that incorporates genetic and genomic tools in veterinary practices. This approach can not only further animal health and welfare but also bolster the productivity and economic health of cattle operations, fostering a mutually beneficial relationship between producers and veterinarians.

A GENETIC APPROACH TO REDUCE DYSTOCIA
The Wide-Ranging Impacts of Dystocia

Veterinarians frequently respond to calls for assistance with dystocia, which refers to abnormal or challenging births.[3] The primary factors contributing to dystocia include maternal or fetal disproportion, fetal malpresentation, and dam-related causes (eg, uterine torsion).[4] Heifers are particularly susceptible to dystocia, largely due to maternal or fetal disproportion, as heifers are still growing and their pelvic canals have not yet fully developed to their mature size.[5] Consequently, heifers will struggle more than mature cows to deliver calves of the same size.

On cattle operations, dystocia can be a major factor in calf mortality and the impact goes well beyond the loss of calves at or immediately following birth, setting the stage for enduring health challenges.[6] During a difficult birth, calves are stressed and may suffer from hypoxemia, a condition where oxygen deprivation occurs due to umbilical cord constriction or chest compression during delivery. This lack of oxygen can leave calves weak, impairing their ability to stand and nurse promptly. As a direct consequence, their ability to effectively absorb vital immunoglobulins from colostrum is compromised. This reduction in immunity acquisition (ie, failure of passive transfer) leaves dystocia-affected calves more susceptible to a range of subsequent health problems, including scours, navel ill, and pneumonia.[7]

Additionally, the physical strain of dystocia can severely affect the dam, causing trauma that may range from soft tissue damage to more severe conditions such as nerve paralysis or skeletal damage. This not only affects the immediate health of the dam but can also lead to prolonged fertility issues, manifesting as increased days open and diminished reproductive capacity.[8] The economic implications resulting from the cumulative impacts of dystocia are significant, underlining the critical need for effective management and preventative strategies in cattle operations.

The Genetic Solution: Calving Ease Traits

Genetic selection for calving ease traits offers a strategic approach to reducing dystocia incidence in cattle. The calving ease direct (CE or CED) expected progeny difference (EPD) is an effective and proven tool for selecting sires to breed with first-calf heifers.[9] An EPD is an objective estimate of genetic merit of an animal based on an animal's pedigree, individual phenotype and those of its relatives, as well as progeny information (once available).[10] CED, quantified as a probability percentage, estimates the likelihood of a sire's offspring being born without assistance when he is bred to heifers. A higher CED value indicates a greater probability of unassisted births, making it a highly desirable trait in sire selection.[9]

CED incorporates multiple sources of phenotypic information, including birth-weights and more importantly, calving scores, as part of a multi-trait genetic evaluation.[9] Calving scores are a numerical scale corresponding with the level of difficulty required to birth the calf. The scale ranges from 1 to 5, with 1 indicating no assistance, 2 indicating some assistance, 3 indicating mechanical assistance, 4 indicating a cesarean section (C-section), and 5 indicating an abnormal presentation. CED significantly improves upon the previous selection method that focused solely on birth weight (BW), which is a trait that is unfavorably correlated with growth traits and maternal calving ease. CED is a more complete evaluation and provides a more accurate prediction of a bull's influence on dystocia rates without directly compromising other economically important traits.[11]

In the selection of sires for producing replacement females, it is essential to also factor in maternal calving ease (CEM or MCE), which estimates the ease with which a sire's daughters will calve. It is important to note that CED and CEM exhibit a small, negative genetic correlation. In other words, there exists an antagonistic relationship between these traits, so as one trait increases, the other decreases.[9] Therefore, balanced consideration of both CED and CEM is imperative when selecting the sires of potential replacement females. This example underscores the importance of selecting the appropriate evaluation tool based on the specific breeding objectives.

Given the variability across cattle operations, there is no universally applicable threshold for calving ease traits that suits all contexts. However, producers can tailor their breeding strategies by analyzing historic calving records and collaborating with their veterinarians to establish custom benchmarks for their operations. This process helps identify the optimal balance of calving ease traits specific to their herd's needs. Strategically reducing dystocia has multiple benefits. It not only significantly improves calving outcomes and calf health, aligning with the core objectives of veterinary care, but also has the potential to reduce labor and feed costs under certain scenarios. Calving ease is just 1 illustrative example of the importance of veterinarians to be well-versed in selection tools that offer tangible advantages for animal health. By doing so, they will be better positioned to initiate and facilitate discussions with their clients toward the effective adoption of these tools, which can have long-lasting benefits for the animals and their producers.

Strategic Sire Selection: Calving Success on a Ranch in Southwest Kansas

Reflecting on the case of a commercial ranch in southwest Kansas, one can see a clear example of how strategic and disciplined sire selection can lead to significant reductions in dystocia rates and yield economic advantages (R. Spare, personal communication). In 1995, this operation faced a daunting challenge with a dystocia rate exceeding 35%, necessitating caesarian sections in 10% of cases.

At that time, the calving season demanded rigorous and resource-intensive monitoring efforts and stretched between 60 and 70 days. Heifers (130 head) were calved in a dry lot, which imposed a considerable investment in feed. The ranch also allocated significant labor resources, employing 3 full-time laborers alongside a ranch manager, to closely monitor the heifers for any signs of calving difficulty at 2-hour intervals. Despite these exhaustive measures, the ranch still experienced significant calf mortality, with losses exceeding 10% for calves past the age of 70 days.

The ranch's previous breeding strategy was to use Angus and crossbred bulls with low-birth-weight phenotypes for breeding first-calf heifers. Facing such significant calving difficulties, this ranch collaborated with its veterinarian to find solutions for enhancing herd health and minimizing calf stress. The ranch began to explore the potential of using EPDs to tackle calving difficulties. Initially focusing on BW, the ranch later shifted to emphasize CED as it became available, recognizing its superior predictive value for calving ease. Three decades later, the ranch has refined its selection criteria to embrace a multi-trait strategy that not only prioritizes calving ease, selecting sires within the top 5% of the breed for CED, but also targets growth and carcass quality.

This comprehensive selection approach has yielded remarkable results. In 2023, the ranch achieved dystocia rates and calf mortality of less than 1%, and the calving season has been streamlined to just 45 days. This reduction in calving difficulties has significantly streamlined calving operations, minimizing the need for extensive resources. Currently, the ranch oversees 115 heifers across 800 acres of pasture, enabling them to graze on natural forage with supplementation. This method of range-calving heifers offers numerous health benefits for the calves, including a cleaner environment with lower microbial contamination and reduced disease transmission. Additionally, range-calving fosters a stronger bond between calf and dam, which further enhances colostrum absorption rates.[12] Moreover, the labor requirements for monitoring have been drastically reduced, now requiring only 1.5 employees who perform checks twice daily. This transformation highlights the efficacy of strategic sire selection based on EPDs in enhancing calving efficiency, improving calf survival, and optimizing labor and resource allocation.

INTEGRATING VETERINARY EXPERTISE WITH GENOMIC INSIGHTS FOR ENHANCED DECISION-MAKING

Historically, cattle production was based on the premise of minimizing inputs and reducing losses, with fed cattle pricing before the 1990s being based on averages that neglected individual quality. Consequently, this approach often undervalued high-quality cattle while over-valuing lower-quality cattle.[13] Therefore, selection primarily focused on phenotype, especially weight. Even today with predictive technologies available, when cattle are sold through local sale barns or video auctions, there is a lack of objective description of expected performance based on genetic merit. Instead, the price received is still primarily driven by weight, along with sex, breed makeup, conditions, lot size, health, and other phenotypic traits.[14]

In the 1990s, the cattle industry shifted toward recognizing and rewarding quality differences through value-based marketing, introducing a system to assign premiums or discounts based on specific quality attributes.[13] This "grid" system encouraged producers to make informed decisions and improve herd quality significantly.

Concurrent with the shift toward value-based marketing, EPD's provided through breed associations became an increasingly valuable tool for seedstock producers, offering a reliable prediction of an animal's genetic potential.[15] Initially, commercial cow-calf producers, lacking direct access to EPDs, depended on seedstock suppliers to incorporate these selection tools into their operations. This reliance was grounded in the trust that seedstock suppliers were using the selection tools effectively ensuring the bulls they provided would enhance the genetic quality of the commercial cow herds. Today, with advancements in genomic technology, both seedstock and commercial producers can access comprehensive data for more informed, data-driven decisions.

Genomic Era in Beef

While the idea of selecting cattle based on their deoxyribonucleic acid (DNA) (ie, genomic selection) was first introduced in 2001,[16] it was not until the first bovine genome was sequenced in 2006[17] that genotyping platforms could be made commercially available. Since then, there has been exponential growth in the understanding of the bovine genome as it relates to performance, as well as the availability of genomic technology. More importantly, there has been a corresponding decrease in the cost of genotyping, making the technology affordable and applicable to producers of all sizes.

Genomic selection is enabled by estimating the effects of single nucleotide polymorphisms (SNPs). SNPs are common variations in DNA that occur at a specific position in the genome. The SNP effects are estimated by analyzing animals that have been both genotyped and phenotyped for specific traits (forming the training population). By utilizing an individual's SNP genotypes in conjunction with the previously estimated SNP effects, molecular breeding values (MBV) for any individual with genotype data can be calculated.[18] In other words, by analyzing the relationship between SNPs and the performance data from a reference group, the influence of these SNPs can be estimated. This information then enables the prediction of the genetic potential of other animals that have been genotyped but were not included in the original study group.

Despite the proven potential of these technologies to enhance profitability, their uptake in the beef industry lags behind that seen in other competing meat industries, often due to lack of exposure and understanding of their significant economic advantages.[19] Veterinarians, as highly trusted advisors, and frequent consultants for beef producers,[1] are uniquely positioned to bridge the gap in the adoption of genomic technologies within the beef industry.

Genomic Data: Different Levels of Investment

Producers have a range of investment options in genomic technology, and the levels vary according to their specific role in the beef supply chain. The quality and depth of genomic insights producer gains directly correlate with the extent of their investment in these technologies (**Table 1**), underscoring the importance of strategic investment in genomics to maximize the potential benefits for their operations.

Parentage verification

The entry level for using genomic technology in beef cattle is verifying an individual's sire and dam through parentage. While parentage was initially made available using a handful of short tandem repeats within the bovine genome, the creation of SNP technology made it much more accurate and affordable. Today, the International Society for Animal Genetics approves the use of 200 SNP for comparison from parent(s) to progeny to verify and accept that the sire and dam reported are the most likely parents of an individual.[20]

Correctly identifying the parents of an animal has substantial benefits. For seedstock producers, it can verify the accuracy of pedigrees being reported for genetic evaluations, ensuring bulls and females are marketed accurately.[19,21] Additionally, parentage verification enables producers to resolve uncertainties between artificial insemination and natural sire contributions when birth dates are inconclusive and also to effectively manage multiple sire breeding pastures.[21] This capability is particularly valuable given research findings that in multiple sire breeding pastures, certain bulls are significantly more prolific, siring a greater number of calves than their counterparts in the same pasture.[22] The ability to verify the sire of calves also enables the identification of bulls that (1) have a disproportionate impact on profitability, (2) may contribute to birthing difficulties or carry genetic defects, and (3) that produce superior (or inferior) offspring. It should be noted that parentage verification is often included as

Table 1
Comparison of input requirements and outputs across different genetic and genomic selection tools

		Selection Tool			
		Parentage	MBV	EPD	GE-EPD
	Industry Sector	Seedstock or Commercial	Commercial	Seedstock or Commercial[a]	Seedstock or Commercial[a]
INPUT	Overall level of input	Low	Low	Moderate - High	High
	DNA sample	Yes	Yes	No	Yes
	Data required	Potential sire(s) and dam(s)	None	Pedigree and phenotype(s)	Pedigree and phenotype(s)
	Level of investment in genomic technology	$	$$	n/a	$$
OUTPUT	Deliverable	Qualified sire and dam	Commercial genomic profile	Genetic predictions for ERTs	Genomic predictions for ERTs
	Accuracy	High	Moderate	Moderate - High	High

Abbreviations: EPD, expected progeny difference; ERT, economically relevant trait; GE-EPD, genomically enhanced EPD; MBV, molecular breeding value; n/anonapplicable.

[a] These services were traditionally provided by breed associations on registered animals. Today, they can also be provided through commercial genetic evaluation services.

part of the broader genomic services available to producers, as described in the following.

Genomically enhanced expected progeny difference

The most accurate predictions of genetic merit are provided in the form of genomically enhanced EPDs (GE-EPD), available to registered cattle of multiple breeds through their respective breed associations. The first estimates of genetic merit in American Angus cattle were traditional EPDs published in 1974.[15] It was not until late 2009 that genomic selection tools became available to cattle producers. However, the journey toward widespread adoption of genomic testing has been gradual. By 2014, only 7 beef-breed associations had amassed genotypes on more than 1000 animals within their databases, which is considered the entry point for generating reliable GE-EPDs.[19] Today, the American Angus Association reports that over half of the 300000 animals registered every year are accompanied by a genomic test, and as of July 2021, they have more than 1 million genotypes in their database.[15]

Using traditional EPDs, young sires were often considered 'unproven' until a sufficient number of progeny records were reported to validate their genetic merit, often delaying their selection as sires. Today, the addition of genomic information to the genetic evaluation allows for increased confidence in the prediction, which is reflected in an increase in accuracy. In fact, recent research suggests that for traits with high heritability, such as growth characteristics, the genotypic data can offer more accurate predictions than performance records alone.[23] Additionally, these recent data demonstrate that genotyped American Angus animals, even without performance or the progeny data, now achieve a level of genetic prediction accuracy comparable to having 8 or more progeny records for all evaluated traits. Notably, for specific traits such as yearling weight, BW, CED, weaning weight, and milk, the accuracy surpasses that of 20 progeny equivalents.[23]

The increased accuracy significantly mitigates operational risks for commercial herds that purchase bulls with GE-EPDs. It increases reliability over traditional EPDs, which are based primarily on the average genetic potential of an animal's parents, and ensures a more predictable breeding outcome.[19] Overall, genotyping has the potential to generate considerable value within the entire beef industry from the seedstock producer to the end product consumer.[21]

Commercial genomic testing

The prediction of quantitative traits, using a limited number of DNA markers was first commercialized in the 1990s. However, it was not until the early 2000s that true commercial genomic predictions in cattle became available.[24] Unlike seedstock breeders, commercial producers often lack incentives to collect comprehensive data points and information, primarily because they do not have direct access to genetic evaluations through breed associations. As a result, initially most genomic testing options available to commercial producers were based solely on the DNA of the animal, providing a useful but limited snapshot of genetic potential. While the initial validation trials of these commercial genomic tests did not meet the industry's high expectations,[25] significant advancements have been made since then.[24,26] Over the past 2 decades, advancements in technology and a deepened understanding of the cattle genome have significantly improved genomic selection for commercial cattle.

Today, commercial producers have 2 genomic prediction options available. The first, more extensive, option involves generating commercial EPDs by reporting pedigree and phenotype information to a genetic evaluation provider. In other words, if a commercial producer wishes to have similar information provided to them as a seedstock breeder, it is now possible but demands significant time and data collection efforts to be successful.

The second option involves simply submitting a DNA sample from an animal to obtain MBVs, which are estimated solely from the animal's genetic makeup. The current commercial products available include predictions for numerous traits of economic importance to a commercial producer, from calving ease to marbling. In a recent study, researchers found that for 6 traits evaluated by a commercial product, the MBV of the dam, while not perfect, had a significant effect on the calf's performance for that trait.[24] It was suggested that the discrepancies present were due to Mendelian sampling and the fact that only half of the DNA of the calf is accounted for in the MBV. Moreover, it is important to understand that genetic predictions aim to estimate the average performance of a group of progeny relative to the population average, rather than predicting individual animal performance.

Continued research into the accuracy of commercial genomic predictions is essential. Currently, the application of genomic testing in commercial operations is seen as a promising tool, albeit underutilized. If further studies validate the precision of these genomic predictions for key traits, it could motivate producers to embrace this technology more broadly. Such a shift would not only enhance genetic progress but also elevate profitability by enabling more precise selection of replacement females[24] and the marketing of steer calves with superior genetic merit.

Leveraging genomics and veterinary knowledge for strategic decisions

Access to more comprehensive data on each animal through veterinary insights and genomic data can significantly enhance the decision-making process for producers. Genomic technologies, by identifying parentage and genetic merit, offer insights into an animal's value. Such insights were not feasible just 2 decades ago. This technology serves as a versatile tool, to both add value and reduce risk across various industry sectors.

At the seedstock level, the industry has become comfortable with GE-EPDs and they recognize the value this information brings toward the marketing of an animal. There is an added value to the sale price of seedstock bulls or heifers because GE-EPDs lower the risk for buyers by providing a more accurate representation of an animal's genetic potential. GE-EPDs also reduce the risk for seedstock suppliers by ensuring selected animals align with the breeding objectives of their buyers and will represent their seedstock program effectively when they move on to their next home.

While genomic technology in the cow-calf sector is not entirely new, its application remains relatively novel. The core aim remains to provide producers with objective data, enabling them to evaluate all marketing strategies before weaning. For instance, determining the genetic potential of replacement heifers provides critical selection criteria, previously unknown to producers. Understanding whether a heifer has more reproductive potential within the herd or growth potential for feedlot performance is crucial, especially with the ongoing success and premiums for feeder cattle genetically verified for superior carcass quality.[27] Today, producers can add value to their feeder calves by offering purchasers animals backed by data, supporting their potential for performance on a value-based grid.

Consider a ranch in the panhandle of Oklahoma managing 70 mature cows and 30 heifers (R. Spare, personal communication). This ranch employs comprehensive herd health management and nutrition strategies in collaboration with its veterinarian. Moreover, the ranch has invested in genomic technology, ensuring that genomic predictions are available for all females and calves to guide selection, breeding, and marketing decisions. The breeding program includes AI of all cows and heifers, followed by exposure to a natural service sire for 75 and 45 days, respectively. At 90 days post-insemination, the ranch works closely with its veterinarian to conduct ultrasounds for pregnancy confirmation and fetal sex determination.

By integrating genomic insights with pregnancy and fetal sex data, the ranch can make targeted marketing decisions aimed at optimizing economic outcomes (**Fig. 1**).

1. Retain bred females: Heifers and cows (<6 years-old) bred early that align with the ranch's breeding goals are kept in the herd.
2. Market bred females: Heifers and cows bred late or not meeting the ranch's breeding objectives, are marketed with genomic data.
3. Market all cows older than 6 years, regardless of breeding status, with genomic information.
4. Feed-out open heifers: Retain open heifers and place them on feed for direct market beef sales through the ranch.
5. Market bull calves: Develop bull calves that meet the ranch's phenotypic and genetic standards, and market them as herd bulls after a breeding soundness evaluation, with the genomic data.
6. Feed-out male calves: Direct male calves that do not fit the ranch criteria to a commercial feed yard for beef production, marketed through the ranch.

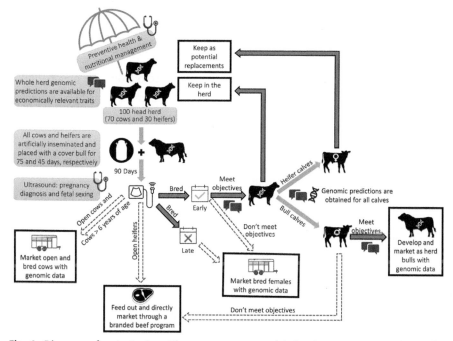

Fig. 1. Diagram of a strategic cattle management model that integrates genomic insights with pregnancy and fetal sex data, to guide selection and marketing choices for enhanced economic returns. Several decision pathways are provided so that every animal is directed through a specific value-added market. The steps that require traditional veterinary skills are denoted by stethoscopes (*purple*). Additionally, conversation bubbles (*purple*) highlight critical points where veterinarians with knowledge of genomic selection can engage with producers, guiding them toward genetic improvement and increased profitability. Arrows with solid outlines (*blue filled*) represent pathways for animals that meet the operation's criteria; arrows with dashed outlines (*red*) represent pathways for animals that do not.

In this real-world example, every animal is directed through a specific value-added market based on high-value services provided by the veterinarian combined with genomic information.

SUMMARY

In an era where veterinary practices are continuously evolving, embracing genetic tools is becoming increasingly vital. As veterinarians deepen their understanding of genetic selection tools, they can substantially enhance the services they offer to producers, from improving animal health to enhancing breeding and marketing decisions. Such expertise in genetics allows veterinarians to provide objective, science-based consultation. Innovative veterinarians can integrate their skills with genetic insights to increase profitability for their clients by boosting the value of their animals through targeting selection and breeding strategies and enabling strategic, value-based marketing options.

Veterinarians, often seen as primary influencers in health and nutritional management, are now poised to become instrumental in increasing adoption of genetic selection tools, helping to optimize animal health, reduce risk, and improve economic outcomes. By embracing genetic selection tools, veterinarians can not only facilitate genetic progress in herds but also open up potential new revenue streams for their practices and clients. The modern beef producer, entrepreneurial in spirit, seeks services that surpass conventional veterinary offerings. These services are more consultative, transforming the veterinarian into a critical asset for the producer. To align the proper tools with the goals of their producers, a veterinarian must facilitate discussions to understand the objectives of the producer and communicate recommendations effectively to help reach them.

Ultimately, by understanding the diverse production sectors and the genetic tools available, veterinarians can be proactive advisors to enhance animal health, product quality, and marketing strategies, transcending the traditional role of crisis management.

CLINICS CARE POINTS

- Proactive advisory role: Provide added value by actively serving as trusted advisors on comprehensive herd health management, including nutrition and genetics.
- Knowledge of selection tools: Engage in ongoing professional development to become familiar with genetic and genomic selection tools, especially concerning traits that directly impact animal health, such as calving ease.
- Utilize CED: Encourage clients to utilize the CED EPD to minimize the incidence of dystocia.
- Integration of the genomic data: Facilitate client discussions about integrating the genomic data with traditional veterinary insights, to tailor herd management and marketing practices to optimize economic returns.

DISCLOSURE

The authors have nothing to disclose.

FUNDING

Mueller was supported by the Kansas Agricultural Experiment Station and U.S. Department of Agriculture (USDA), National Institute of Food and Agriculture Grant no. 2021-67034-3515.

REFERENCES

1. U.S. Department of Agriculture (USDA). Beef 2017 report 1: beef cow-calf management practices in the United States. NAHMS Beef Cow-Calf Studies; 2020. Available at: https://www.aphis.usda.gov/animal_health/nahms/beefcowcalf/downloads/beef2017/Beef2017_dr_PartI.pdf. [Accessed 15 February 2024].
2. U.S. Department of Agriculture (USDA). Beef 2007–08 Part IV: Reference of Beef Cow-calf Management Practices in the United States. In: NAHMS beef cow-calf studies. 2010. Available at: https://www.aphis.usda.gov/animal_health/nahms/beefcowcalf/downloads/beef0708/Beef0708_dr_PartIV_1.pdf. [Accessed 15 February 2024].
3. Hilton WM. Practical OB tips. In: AABP conference proceedings. 2018. Available at: https://bovine-ojs-tamu.tdl.org/AABP/article/view/3268. [Accessed 15 February 2024].
4. Zaborski D, Grzesiak W, Szatkowska I, et al. Factors Affecting Dystocia in Cattle. Reprod Domest Anim 2009;44(3):540–51.
5. Waldner C. Cow attributes, herd management and environmental factors associated with the risk of calf death at or within 1 h of birth and the risk of dystocia in cow-calf herds in Western Canada. Livest Sci 2014;163.
6. Lombard JE, Garry FB, Tomlinson SM, et al. Impacts of Dystocia on Health and Survival of Dairy Calves. J Dairy Sci 2007;90(4):1751–60.
7. Godden SM, Lombard JE, Woolums AR. Colostrum Management for Dairy Calves. Vet Clin North Am Food Anim Pract 2019;35(3):535–56.
8. Boakari YL, Ali HE-S. Management to Prevent Dystocia. In: Hopper RM, editor. Bovine reproduction. 2nd edition. Hoboken: Wiley-Blackwell; 2021. p. 590–6.
9. Rolf MM. Genetic Correlations and Antagonisms. In: eBeef. 2019. Available at: https://beef-cattle.extension.org/genetic-correlations-and-antagonisms/. [Accessed 15 February 2024].
10. Spangler M. EPD Basics and Definitions. In: eBeef. 2019. Available at: https://beef-cattle.extension.org/epd-basics-and-definitions/. [Accessed 15 February 2024].
11. Bennett GL, Thallman RM, Snelling WM, et al. Genetic changes in beef cow traits following selection for calving ease. Transl Anim Sci 2021;5(1).
12. Nevard RP, Pant SD, Broster JC, et al. Maternal Behavior in Beef Cattle: The Physiology, Assessment and Future Directions-A Review. Vet Sci 2022;10(1).
13. Peel DS, Anderson J. How We Got Here: A Brief History of Cattle and Beef Markets. In: Feedlot magazine. 2022. Available at: https://www.feedlotmagazine.com/news/industry_news/how-we-got-here-a-brief-history-of-cattle-and-beef-markets/article_1fe3c56c-6739-11ec-a5bb-2b72c548a8a4.html. [Accessed 7 February 2024].
14. Dethloff N, Bir C, Holcomb R, et al. Cattle Marketing Plans: Traditional vs. Direct to Consumer. In: OSU extension. 2023. Available at: https://extension.okstate.edu/fact-sheets/cattle-marketing-plans-traditional-vs-direct-to-consumer.html. [Accessed 7 February 2024].
15. Retallick K, Lu D, Garcia A, et al. Genomic selection in the US: where it has been and where it is going?. In: Proceedings of 12th WCGALP. 2022. Available at: . [Accessed 7 February 2024].
16. Meuwissen THE, Hayes BJ, Goddard ME. Prediction of Total Genetic Value Using Genome-Wide Dense Marker Maps. Genetics 2001;157(4):1819–29.
17. Liu Y, Qin X, Song X-ZH, et al. Bos taurus genome assembly. BMC Genom 2009;10(1):180.

18. Meuwissen T, Hayes B, Goddard M. Accelerating Improvement of Livestock with Genomic Selection. Annu Rev Anim Biosci 2013;1(1):221–37.
19. Rolf MM, Decker JE, McKay SD, et al. Genomics in the United States beef industry. Livest Sci 2014;166:84–93.
20. International Society for Animal Genetics (ISAG). Guidelines for cattle parentage verification based on SNP markers. In: ISAG conference proceedings. 2012. Available at: https://www.isag.us/Docs/Guideline-for-cattle-SNP-use-for-parentage-2012.pdf. [Accessed 7 February 2024].
21. Bullock D, Spangler M, Van Eenennaam AL, et al. Delivering genomics technology to the beef industry. In: National beef cattle evaluation consortium white paper. 2012. Available at: https://www.nbcec.org/topics/WhitePaperGenomicsTechnology.pdf. [Accessed 7 February 2024].
22. Drake DJ, Weber KL, Van Eenennaam AL. What are herd bulls accomplishing in multiple sire breeding pastures. In: Proceedings, applied reproductive strategies in beef cattle. 2011. Available at: https://ucanr.edu/sites/UCCE_LR/files/155931.pdf. [Accessed 7 February 2024].
23. Miller S. Genomic selection in beef cattle creates additional opportunities for embryo technologies to meet industry needs. Reprod Fertil Dev 2022;35(2):98–105.
24. Arisman BC, Rowan TN, Thomas JM, et al. Evaluation of Zoetis GeneMax Advantage genomic predictions in commercial *Bos taurus* Angus cattle. Livest Sci 2023;274:105266.
25. Van Eenennaam AL, Li J, Thallman RM, et al. Validation of commercial DNA tests for quantitative beef quality traits. J Anim Sci 2007;85(4):891–900.
26. Weber KL, Drake DJ, Taylor JF, et al. The accuracies of DNA-based estimates of genetic merit derived from Angus or multibreed beef cattle training populations. J Anim Sci 2012;90(12):4191–202.
27. Brink T. Genetics valued over hide color: Feedlot Managers Desire Change in the Feeder Cattle Market. In: Red Angus association - white paper. 2022. Available at: https://redangus.org/genetics-valued-over-hide-color-feedlot-managers-desire-change-in-the-feeder-cattle-market/. [Accessed 7 February 2024].

Sampling and Laboratory Logistics

How to Collect DNA Samples and Overview of Techniques for Laboratory Analysis

Susanne Hinkley, DVM, PhD[a],*, Richard G. Tait Jr, MS, PhD, PAS[b]

KEYWORDS

- Genetic defect • DNA • Genotyping • Sampling • Genetic selection

KEY POINTS

- High-quality sample collection is a fundamental requirement to provide insightful genotyping results to a client.
- Ideal sample collection devices ease the sample collection process on farm, are rapid to deploy on individual animals during routine animal processing, provide a means to store the sample for shipment, and facilitate processing at the genotyping laboratory. All are important features when choosing a sample collection system.
- Knowing the genotypic status of animals allows more informed decisions and usage of animals from families which would have historically been avoided because of the risk of unfavorable attributes (eg, carrier of a recessive defect).

INTRODUCTION

Understanding genetic control of a variety of traits over the past several decades has evolved from an understanding and appreciation of tracking relevant families and pedigrees to manage risk of an unwanted genetic condition (eg, dwarfism) and/or increasing genetic progress for several economically relevant traits at the same time to using genomics to perform these activities more directly. Genomics have allowed more explicit characterization of the genetic status of individual animals, and this is very important for managing risk. Rather than completely avoiding a pedigree that has been identified as a carrier of a recessive defect, now frequently the genetic status can be tested, and it can be determined which descendants carry the mutant allele and which descendants carry the wildtype alleles and thus are free from the defect.

---

[a] Clinical Diagnostics, Neogen Genomics, 4131 North 48th Street, Lincoln, NE 68504, USA;
[b] Genetics Product Development, Neogen Genomics, 4131 North 48th Street, Lincoln, NE 68504, USA
* Corresponding author.
E-mail address: shinkley@neogen.com

Vet Clin Food Anim 40 (2024) 381–398
https://doi.org/10.1016/j.cvfa.2024.05.003
vetfood.theclinics.com

Furthermore, for dominant traits the animal's phenotype is not informative on the genetic configuration (heterozygous or homozygous for dominant version of the gene), and it is, therefore, valuable to know the genetic status. For instance, for the dominant traits of black coat color or polledness in cattle, the phenotype indicates that the animal is either heterozygous or homozygous for the trait. There is potentially a significant difference in the value of an animal homozygous for the trait, passing on that trait to all its offspring, compared to an animal heterozygous for the trait, passing it on to only half of its offspring. Therefore, genomic testing and understanding the actual genotype of an animal for a variety of traits, conditions, and favorable or unfavorable genetic potential is a tool being increasingly implemented across North America and around the world. This article highlights the importance of collecting a good sample from an animal of interest to ensure relevant data are returned to the producer client for their decision-making.

BEST PRACTICES OF SAMPLE COLLECTION IN THE FIELD TO ENSURE SUBMISSION OF GOOD-QUALITY SAMPLES
Getting Started

Sample collection for disease diagnostics is a major part of clinical veterinary practice. Best practices for sample collection for genomic testing are not significantly different, in that submission of a high-quality sample is much more likely to return a useful result than submission of a low-quality sample. All samples sent to the genomic testing laboratory are entered into a laboratory information management system (LIMS). This system tracks arrival of the sample and all steps of processing and testing it is subjected to. Therefore, it is essential that the initial information is correct, starting with the on-farm identification of the animal sampled. Accurate animal records, with permanent well-legible or barcoded scannable ear tags, electronic radio frequency identification (RFID) ear tags, or other reliable means of unique identification should be present. Appropriate restraint of the animal is important so that a full-size sample can be collected without the animal being able to jerk away. Ideally, sample collection should be into a barcoded sample collection device. To minimize animal identification and collection errors when sampling many animals, capture of the animal identification (ID) for each device should be at (with a second person), or immediately following, sample collection. When writing down animal IDs by hand, for example, on the cardboard holder for Allflex tissue sampling unit (TSU) devices (Merck & Co., Inc. Rahway, NJ), care must be taken to write legibly and orient the writing correctly (not upside down; **Fig. 1**). Additionally, the pen ink must be allowed to dry so writing does not smear. When devices are used that are not barcoded, for example, blood tubes, the animal ID must be written on the sampling device. Any smearing of numbers or letters, distorted and illegible characters or unclear orientation of the numbers, specifically for 1, 6, 8, and 9, will all be factors that will slow down the accessioning process in the laboratory and allow for errors in animal identification. The simple strategy of placing a small dot at the end of a numerical ID indicates the orientation that ID is to be read and facilitates correct transfer of IDs into the laboratory database. When labeling is done correctly, the accessioning process can be accomplished efficiently and correctly. The more samples the laboratory routinely processes, the more important it is to streamline the individual steps of those processes as much as possible.

Sample devices that are barcoded can be read efficiently and correctly on the farm and in the laboratory upon receipt, when the accessioning process transfers the sample ID into electronic format and a virtual place for the sample is created in the LIMS. It

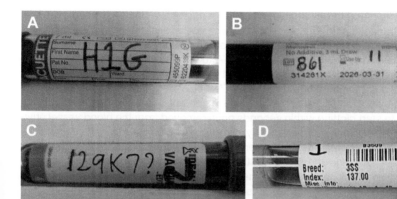

Fig. 1. Examples of labeling on blood tubes. (*A*) No barcode but well-legible. (*B*) Correct orientation of writing so numbers cannot be read upside down (861 vs 198). (*C*) Legible but questionable farm records. (*D*) Preprinted labels, with barcode.

is, therefore, very helpful for the laboratory to receive an electronic manifest (sample list) with a list of barcodes and the respective animal ID in Excel or even Word format. That information can be verified against the barcode scans of all samples physically present in the laboratory. All duplicates or extra samples unaccounted for in the sample list can thereby be identified and the customer notified.

Choosing the Right Sample Type and Sample Collection Device

Sample quality is essential for successful processing of samples in the laboratory and subsequent delivery of quality data and results that are worth the investment to the customer. In turn, a sample can only be of good quality if (1) the sample matrix is suitable for the purpose; (2) there is sufficient quantity/volume of sample; and (3) sample integrity has not been compromised.

For sampling live animals for the purpose of genotyping, there are several options, both for sample types and collection devices. Different sample types will yield different amounts of DNA, depending on the number and density of the nucleated cells the tissues or body fluids contain. It is also noteworthy that, if several tests are requested for a single sample (eg, parentage and specific traits such as milk proteins or tenderness), the required amount of DNA will be higher than, if only, a single test (eg, GGP Bovine 100K) is requested.

Likewise, some sample collection devices are useful for certain sample sizes or animal sizes and some sample types are easier to process than others. Depending on the number of tests requested for one sample, more DNA might be required. Some sample collection devices are convenient and efficient to work within the field but require intensive, hands-on protocols for processing. All in all, when deciding what collection device and what sample type to use, one should consider the ease and efficiency of sample collection in the field, the cost of the collection device and efficiency, speed, and cost to process the resulting sample in the laboratory. The following list discusses a variety of sample matrices the Neogen Genomics laboratory has received and processed successfully.

Sample matrices, live animals/ante mortem
Whole blood. Traditionally, whole blood is widely used, and the presence of numerous white blood cells generally ensures adequate DNA yields from this sample

type. For whole blood to be useable, however, it must have been collected in ethylenediaminetetraacetic acid (EDTA)-coated tubes (readily available from several manufacturers and through veterinary supply distributors), indicated by the purple-colored top. Additionally, once collected into the EDTA tube, the blood must immediately be mixed with the EDTA, gently by inversion, not by shaking. If the blood is collected in a syringe first and then transferred to the EDTA tube, one must work very fast. Otherwise, there is a substantial risk of microclot development because of the propensity of whole blood to start clotting within seconds once removed from the blood vessel environment. Onset of clotting is particularly fast in avian blood. While the presence of moderate amounts of microclots is tolerable for laboratory processing, completely clotted whole blood and the serum resulting after centrifugation are unsuitable for DNA extraction and will get rejected in the laboratory. Likewise, whole blood samples collected in red top or "tiger" top serum separator tubes get rejected outright for genotyping. This applies to all species.

Another caveat must be mentioned: When genotyping twins in cattle, whole blood is unsuitable as sample type. Dizygotic cattle twins share the chorionic blood supply in utero, so the genetic profile of one twin will always appear "contaminated" with the DNA from the other twin. A clear genetic profile, thereby, cannot be obtained of either animal. In the case of opposite-sex bovine twins, freemartin females will almost always develop. Even though the twinning rate is estimated to be low (less than 6%) in cattle,[1] embryonic or early fetal death of one of the twins may mask the presence of a twin pregnancy altogether. In cases of known twinning, a hair follicle or tissue sample is recommended for genotyping and sample types containing much blood should be avoided. While the freemartin phenomenon in cattle is well documented and extensively studied, there is limited research available on the frequency in sheep and goats. In sheep, multiple births with males and females are fairly common but freemartins appear to be rare.[2,3]

For maintenance of optimal sample quality, whole blood should be stored at refrigerator temperatures and shipped in a temperature-controlled environment, that is, on ice packs in an insulated shipping container. Freezing should be avoided, especially when using glass tubes. Traditional glass tubes are particularly fragile, but even plastic tubes must be secured during shipping to prevent the tubes from jostling in transit. Extra packing material must be added as necessary. Samples in broken tubes are usually rejected for testing due to likely cross contamination and staff safety concerns.

Blood cards. If whole blood samples are unable to be stored, blood cards are an option. Blood cards consist of a filter paper with a thin cardboard front and back, bearing a barcode. Cards are labeled with the animal ID, then whole blood is spotted on the filter paper, soaking into the paper until the spot fills the black circle on the paper. Devices to access the blood vessel (eg, needle or razor blade) must not be shared between animals. A well-spotted blood card will have the circle filled completely (slight overfill will not be a problem) and the blood soaked through to the other side of the paper. Blood cards should be dried at room temperature. Specifically for the purpose of drying, blood card backings provide 2 slots for the top card. The upper one is used for drying position, with the top card and the filter paper slightly bent so they do not touch any other part of the card. The lower slot is used after blood has completely dried for closing the card flat (**Fig. 2**A–D). Well-spotted blood cards generally dry sufficiently within about 12 hours. The blood spot must be completely dry to the touch. Only then can the card be fully closed (using the lower slot), laid flat, and stored at room temperature. Generally, blood cards are barcoded and, thereby, enable a dual

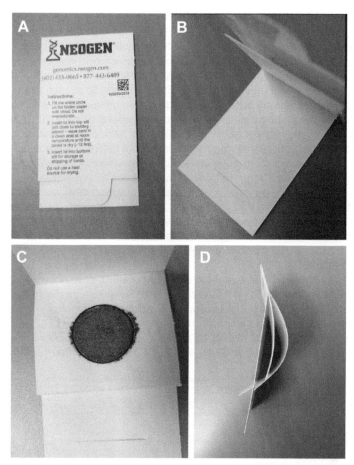

Fig. 2. Blood cards. (*A*) Standard blood card, with instructions. (*B*) Open card showing the 2 slots; upper slot for drying and lower slot for folding flat. (*C*) Blood card spotted correctly. (*D*) Cross-section view of blood card in drying position. (*A*) *With permission from* Dr. Susanne Hinkley, DVM PhD, Director, Clinical Diagnostics, Neogen Genomics.

identification method (barcode plus animal ID) in the laboratory that minimizes identification errors and allows for high-throughput processing via barcode scanning.

Tissues. There are different tissues that are suitable for successful DNA extraction. A notable exception is fat tissues as they contain few cells. Moreover, the fat content of the cells is extremely hydrophobic and does not mix with water-based extraction reagents routinely used in the laboratory. The most convenient and easily collectable tissue in cattle is the skin of the ear, either as punch or fresh ear notch. Tissue punches can be collected in different devices. Punch sizes average 3 to 4 mm in diameter. Commercially available collection devices are marketed with an emphasis on convenience in that they can be stored, even after the sample has been collected, at room temperature. Consequently, they contain either a liquid preservative or other substances (like desiccant) to prevent the collected tissue punch from decaying and thereby becoming unsuitable for DNA extraction. Furthermore, tissue punch containers are barcoded by the manufacturer that enables dual identification methods in the laboratory and allows for high-throughput processing. Examples of widely available tissue collection devices are tissue sampling units (https://www.allflex.global/na/product/tissue-sampling-unit/) or TypiFix devices (https://us.ztags.com/products/livestock-tags/tissue-sampler). Both are available either through genomic testing laboratories directly or through veterinary supplies distributors.

In the ongoing effort to maximize efficiency, laboratories will always prefer a bar-coded vial containing precut, suitably sized, tissue pieces. To access the tissue, vials must be opened individually but automated de-capping makes this step much more efficient and, usually, laboratories have at least some level of automation in place to process standard and widely used tissue collection devices. Automation minimizes human errors and creates efficiency in high-throughput settings, thereby creating savings that can be passed on to customers. For an automation example, see https://www.youtube.com/watch?app=desktop&v=Jpqlch_9dCE.

At the same time, automation is largely intolerant to high variability, and it is the sample submitter's responsibility to follow best practices to minimize such variability (**Fig. 3**A–E). Giving the sample collection devices a good last look to check for the presence of tissue prior to sending the sample(s) to the laboratory (**Fig. 4**) is one of those best practices that all too often gets neglected. Examples of rejected samples are shown in **Fig. 5**.

It must be remembered that an ear tag (standard or RFID) does not necessarily double as tissue collection device. All tissue collection devices require the animal owner or sample submitter to purchase the appropriate applicator.

Fresh tissues cannot be stored at room temperature for any length of time but must be frozen or shipped immediately on ice packs to preserve the quality of the sample. Examples of fresh tissue submissions are fresh ear notches from cattle, pig tails

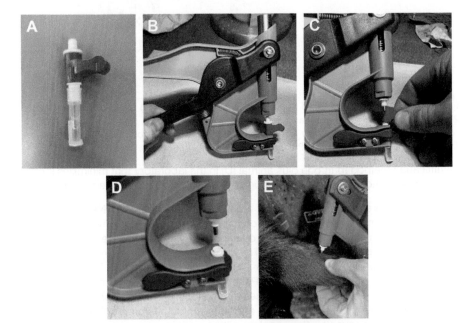

Fig. 3. Correct assembly of Allflex TSU device into the appropriate applicator and sampling of the cattle ear. (*A*) Unused collection device with top punch still attached. (*B*) Locking collection vial into the bottom of the applicator and the top punch into the upper part of the applicator. (*C*) Removal of the spacer to expose the metal punch. (*D*) Applicator and TSU ready for sampling. (*E*) Sampling of a cattle ear. (Allflex®. With permission from Merck & Co., Inc.)

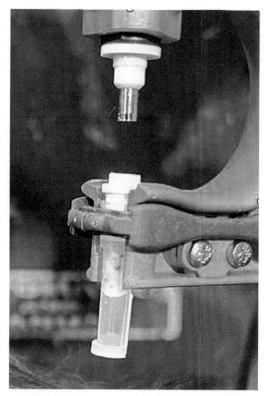

Fig. 4. Successful sampling of the cattle ear. Visible tissue in the vial. Green ball (original seal, visible from the top when vial is unused) now on the bottom of the vial, red plunger pushed all the way in, sealing the top. Top seal is now red.

collected at the time of tail docking and castrating piglets, or fin clips from freshwater fish in aquaculture. If large numbers of samples are to be submitted, storage in the freezer prior to shipping might become a problem, depending on the size of the collection device chosen by the owner. Clean/sterile bags, cups or tubes are all acceptable if they can be closed securely, labeled clearly, and are leak proof. However, any containers chosen will have to be provided (purchased extra) by the owner and they will likely not be barcoded. Another consideration from the perspective of the laboratory is that tissue punchers collect a small but suitably sized sample that can be used as is, but fresh tissue pieces are usually much larger and must be cut to suitable small sizes in the laboratory, a very time-consuming activity that may increase the risk of cross contamination.

Formalin-fixed tissues, unfortunately, are not suitable for submission for genomic testing because formalin damages DNA by random severe fragmentation, base modification, and cross-linkage with itself or proteins.[4] Even though DNA can be readily recovered from those specimens, it is unsuitable for downstream processing of the sample for genotyping.

Hair follicles. Another sample type, convenient for the owner to collect, is hair follicles, primarily for sampling cattle (**Fig. 6**). For collection, a pair of pliers can be used to grab 1 or 2 bunches of hair and pull them out in a manner that the follicles that anchor the hair in the skin remain attached to the hair shaft. Only the follicles contain DNA, the hair shafts

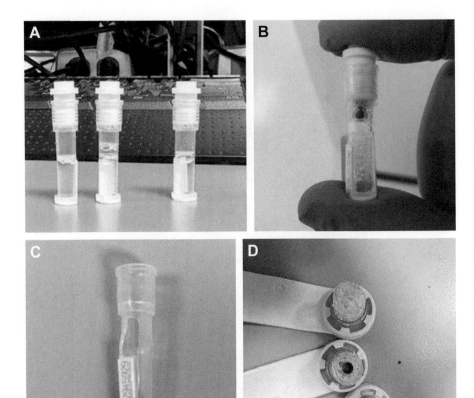

Fig. 5. Samples received in the laboratory that had to be rejected for containing no tissue. (*A*) No green ball visible, faulty device? (*B*) Green ball and red plunger visible. Correct handling of the applicator but missed the tissue of the ear. (*C*) Tissue piece and buffer lost from the vial; vial wall melted. (*D*) TypiFix devices after opening and removal of dry desiccant: missing puncher (top device); no evidence of tissue in the metal puncher piece (2 bottom devices).

do not. For cattle, the best place to sample is the tail switch because tail hair is very thick and coarse and usually has good-sized follicles. In horses, specifically in thoroughbred foals for registration with the Jockey Club, mane hairs are collected. Pig hair can be collected from the body as the body hair is coarse and follicle size is suitable. Altogether, 2 main best practices must be considered for collection. First, ample numbers of hair shafts and their follicles must be collected to enable sufficient DNA yield. The presence of 30 to 40 follicles per sample is preferred. Second, the hair shafts should be fixed in a sampling container such that they all point in one direction, the majority does not overlap, and follicles are clearly visible (**Fig. 7**). The better those practices are considered the easier and faster a laboratory technician can collect the follicles from the hair shafts, 15 to 20 per extraction, using a metal punch. While the upfront purchase price of hair cards may be appealing, they generally carry an upcharge for handling, due to factors that require extra attention and processing time, and may even cause sample rejection. Those factors include (**Fig. 8**) but are not limited to

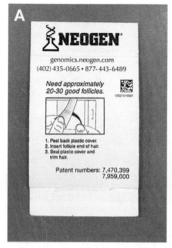
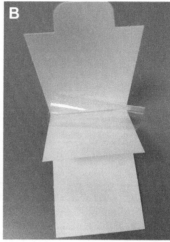

Fig. 6. Specialized hair cards. (*A*) Hair card with instructions. (*B*) Open hair card, showing the support for the hair shafts and the clear sticky sheet to be placed on top of the hair to secure it. (*A*) *With permission from* Dr. Susanne Hinkley, DVM PhD, Director, Clinical Diagnostics, Neogen Genomics.

1. Any amount of contaminating dirt or manure
2. Thin hair shafts with tiny follicles, collected from the body instead of the tail switch
3. White hair
4. Hair from very young animals
5. Hair shafts not pointing in one direction
6. Too many hairs collected and bunched together
7. Not using a specialized hair card with a sticky cover for immobilization of the hair

Swabs. When deciding how to collect suitable samples from small companion animals, primarily dogs and cats, additional considerations come into play. Generally, tissue samples are not a good option, both for cosmetic reasons and because a 3 to

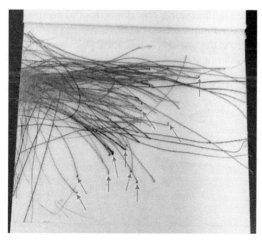

Fig. 7. Excellent hair card. Ample number of hair shafts collected. Sample fanned out, follicles pointing all in one direction, many good follicles present (some indicated by *green arrows*).

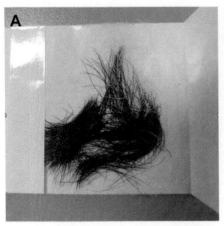
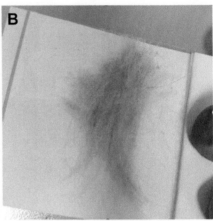

Fig. 8. Examples of poorly collected hair cards, requiring extra effort to process. (*A*) Very thin hair, too many hair shafts collected. Follicles pointing in different directions. Majority of the hair bunched together. (*B*) Too much hair collected, hair shafts pointing in different directions, some dirt, hair bunched together.

4 mm tissue punch like the Allflex TSU would leave an injury of a more significant size, compared to the overall size of the animal. Swab samples have established themselves as convenient and suitable sample type for genomic testing of those companion animals. Although there are many different swab types commercially available, the type primarily validated for genomic testing is a bristle swab (**Fig. 9**), used in the oral cavity.

The bristles on the individual swab are stiff and long enough that they gently scrape and collect enough cells of the oral cavity. Given that the swab head is fairly small, a single package contains 2 swabs, and both must be used to ensure collection of sufficient sample material for successful DNA extraction. A rigorous back-and-forth motion, combined with twisting the swab shaft, is essential to dislodge cells in the oral cavity and collect them on the swab, even if animal owners might hesitate to "injure" their animal. For storage and shipping, these swabs are inserted back into their paper sleeve and held at room temperature. The sleeve for the swabs must have the animal ID written on it. The swabs themselves must be barcoded for identification since there will be no place to write on the swab shaft. Since 2 swabs are recommended for sample collection from the animal, 2 identical barcode stickers are included with the package (**Fig. 10**A, B).

Another swab type is the Genotek PG100 swab that is suitable to sample cells from the nostrils of cattle, sheep, and goats and is also used in the oral cavity for dogs, cats,

Fig. 9. Standard bristle swab.

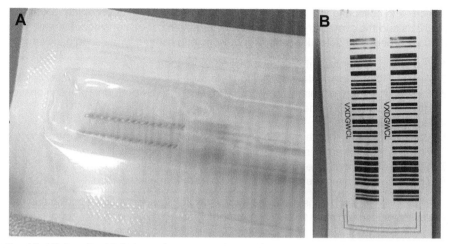

Fig. 10. (*A*) Standard bristle swabs come with 2 swabs per package and (*B*) dual barcode stickers, 1 for the sleeve and 1 for the actual swabs.

and horses. This swab type has a soft spongy head. The PG100 comes with a buffer that preserves the DNA and is also claimed to have bacteriostatic activity, thereby allowing storage of samples at room temperature. The container is barcoded. Conveniently, this sample type can allow for multiple extractions in the laboratory, if necessary.

https://www.dnagenotek.com/US/products/collection-animals/performagene/PG-100.html.

Other swab types, particularly the types routinely used by a veterinary clinician for disease diagnostics, are generally not well validated for DNA extraction from host cells (rather than the suspected pathogens) and should be avoided.

Sample matrices, dead animals/postmortem. As part of a diagnostic routine for a clinician, it may be of interest to investigate whether perinatal mortality on a client's property is the result of a known recessive genetic mutation in that animal, if it is a result of transmissible disease, or may become an important resource for a future genetic investigation.[5] In the situation where an animal has died, collecting whole blood is generally no longer an option, especially not with vacuum-aided blood collection systems. Considering that decomposition will begin very shortly after death, tissues (skin, muscle, or organ tissues) must be collected as soon as possible to maintain integrity of the cells and thereby the DNA. The same is true for collecting hair follicles; one of the first processes of decay after death is hair slipping, indicating decomposition and invasion of bacteria of the skin.[6,7] The rate of autolysis will depend on the environmental temperature, but any decomposition will lower the quality of the sample collected. A best practice would be to collect tissues (skin or muscle) immediately after the animal has been identified to be tested and freeze them to stop further autolysis until submission to the laboratory. Tissues from the abdominal cavity (liver, spleen) should be avoided since bacterial activity after death through leaky intestines will greatly accelerate decomposition. Tissue sampling (primarily muscle) of individual animals in a slaughterhouse (for tracking and tracing purposes) remains a viable option because carcasses get eviscerated and chilled immediately.

Summary of sample type and collection device considerations. Ultimately, the selection of the sampling device varies with the comfort level of the individual handling the devices and collecting the samples. The on-farm availability of appropriate restraining methods and the availability of other people for help must be considered. Ideally, the thought process for selecting sampling devices and sample types should include

1. Availability of appropriate restraint facilities/methods
2. Availability of additional personnel for help
3. Existing inventory of animals for sample collection to be performed on can ensure correct animal IDs at the time of collection
4. Ease of use
5. Cost of the sampling device
6. Following best practices for specific laboratory submissions
7. Storage and shipping temperatures
8. Amount of sample material that can be collected for each device

An overview of such considerations for a variety of sample types and collection devices is provided in **Table 1**.

Submitting Samples to the Laboratory

Once the sample collection has been completed, samples are shipped to the laboratory. Although this might seem like a very simple process, several rules for best practices apply:

1. Include a sample manifest (simple list of all samples with their associated unique barcodes if available and applicable): For accurate on-farm records, each owner/submitter should have that list of samples (either with names, ear tag numbers, or barcodes) saved either on the computer or as a hard copy. Particularly in case a large number of samples are submitted, the manifest should be sent to the laboratory in electronic format.
2. Many laboratories allow and encourage online pre-submission of the samples. With pre-submissions, the sample identifiers are already in the laboratory's LIMS system, and upon arrival the samples only need to be accounted for and checked for duplicates or extra samples. Pre-submission may require the creation of an account with the genotyping laboratory's LIMS system. It is advantageous to work with a representative of the genotyping laboratory to confirm arrival and processing of samples. A representative can also be very helpful to advise on the type of testing that will be most useful to achieve the goal of genotyping on the given operation.
   a. Barcodes on the sample collection devices are very helpful but are not required. The laboratory's Web site will have submission templates, specific for species, breed, and test to be performed, that must be downloaded, completed, and then uploaded to the site.
   b. Including a hardcopy version of the electronic submission form along with the samples in the package is highly recommended, regardless of whether samples are electronically presubmitted or not.
3. Packaging the samples well is essential, particularly for blood tubes. Tubes, even plastic tubes, must be immobilized and not allowed to jostle in the shipping container; otherwise, breakage is likely. Small bubble wrap works well, both for insulation and for cushioning. Crumpled-up newspaper will do as well. Sample tubes can be tethered together with rubber bands for immobilization. Samples should also, collectively, be placed into a plastic bag or several plastic bags and the submission form, if a hard copy is used, should be placed into a separate plastic bag. Thus, in the event of sample breakage, the form does not get soaked and becomes illegible. Blood and fresh tissue samples should be shipped in temperature-controlled

Table 1
Overview of common sample types and collection devices and some of their characteristics

Sample Types	Convenience of Sampling	Sample Container Barcoded	Storage and Shipping Temps	Efficiency of Processing in the Laboratory	Relative Cost	Notes
Allflex Tags	Good, with appropriate restraint	TSU vial, yes	Room temperature	High, automation	$$$	Automated decapper commercially available
Allflex TST	Good, with appropriate restraint	TST vial, yes	Room temperature	Low, no automation	$$$	
Whole Blood	Good, universal training	Probably no	Refrigerated	Moderate	$$	Can go back to, good DNA yield
Hair Card	Good	Hair card, yes	Room temperature	Low	$	Must have enough follicles. Upcharge for processing.
Blood Card	Moderate	Blood card, yes	Room temperature	Moderate	$	DNA yields low to moderate
TypiFix Tag	Good, with appropriate restraint	Sample collection cup, yes	Room temperature	Low, no automation	$$	Dry desiccant: messy
Caisley Tag	Good, with appropriate restraint	Caisley vial, yes	Room temperature	Low, no automation	$$$	Ear tag and tissue collection vial combined
Genotec Swab/PG100	Very good (small animals)	Fluid container, yes	Room temperature	Moderate	$$$$	High-quality liquid preservative
Bristle Swab	Very good (small animals)	Swab sleeve, yes; swabs, no	Room temperature	Moderate	$	Allows for only a single extraction
Fresh Tissue	Primarily postmortem	Probably no	Frozen/refrigerated	Low, must be cut to small size	($) but container not included	Great DNA values, can go back to often if stored frozen
Semen Straws	Livestock: good; small animals: specialized	Probably no	Refrigerated	Low	$$	Can be collected as part of semen quality evaluation

environments, that is, Styrofoam Coolers with ice packs, with next-day delivery service. Sample stabilizing tissue collection devices like Allflex TSUs, Caisley tags, and TypiFix tags can be shipped at room temperature. Shipping by air and the associated high pressures, however, may cause some of the tags to leak so it is advisable to package those vials into plastic bags as well to contain potential leakage. Commercial carriers are hesitant to transport obviously leaked packages, where the liquid contents have soaked through to the outside of the package. It is suggested for submitting veterinarians to stay up to date with shipping requirements for the type of testing to be performed.

4. There are several choices of commercial carriers, including FedEx, UPS, USPS, and DHL. Deciding which carrier to use is most often a matter of convenience and who has the nearest office.
5. All shipping methods and carriers can encounter adverse circumstances and delivery of the samples might be delayed. Timelines for results to be delivered by laboratories will start from the day of arrival at the laboratory, not from the day of shipment.
6. International shipments, for example, from Canada to the United States, are subject to a different set of regulations, including the requirement for an import permit held by the laboratory. Before attempting to ship those samples, the receiving laboratory should be contacted to inquire about the various shipping documents required and what carrier to use. Not all international packages are inspected by customs, but if the package is inspected and incomplete documents are found, the samples will not be allowed to enter the country. This is especially unfortunate for temperature-sensitive samples as the process of customs hold and sample return can take weeks, resulting in significant loss of sample quality.

PROCESSING OF SAMPLES WITHIN THE LABORATORY
Accessioning

Once samples have been accounted for and have been recognized in the laboratory database (LIMS), the processing is initiated, that is, DNA extraction and purification, and the actual genotyping. Before the DNA extraction process can commence, samples need to be organized into the format of processing. Each sample must be identified with a unique laboratory ID that ensures positive identification from the original sample all the way to the report back to the customer. Typically, barcode and animal ID are an essential part of this identification. An overview of the workflow is provided in **Fig. 11**.

DNA Extraction

Different sample types require unique extraction methods and reagents. In the overall process, the first step is organizing, sample sizing and/or transfer, and addition of the appropriate reagents. These steps will require the most specialized attention and extra time if best practices for sample collection and sample submission were not followed. The more uniform the quality of sample collection process and submission is the more likely automation can facilitate preparation of large numbers of samples and enable timely turnaround times. Whether generated by hands-on processes or automated processes, the DNA extracted is ready for the assessment of quantity and quality to verify that it meets the requirements of the ensuing genotyping process.

Processing for Genotyping

While "genotyping" is the summary expression for the activity of determining DNA sequences in various places on the genome, there are subsets of genotyping that vary in their objective. Performing a genotyping test on an animal is initiated for a very specific

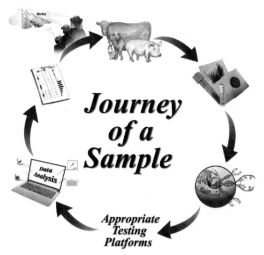

Fig. 11. Journey of a sample (animals, sample collection, DNA extraction, processing and genotyping, data analysis and interpretation, report, decision-making). (*Courtesy of* K. Cottrell, BA, Lincoln, Nebraska.)

objective and generally the results of one test type or objective do not inform another objective for genotyping the animal. Depending on the type of polymorphism or mutation that causes the resultant phenotype, genotyping may represent characterizing (1) microsatellites, also known as short tandem repeats (STRs)[8,9]; (2) single nucleotide polymorphisms (SNPs)[10]; or (3) insertions or deletions:

- Traits may be a key initial attribute to be genotyped on individual animals. In the case of a dominant trait such as polledness or black coat color, the phenotype expressed by the animal would indicate that the animal is either heterozygous or homozygous for that trait. Knowing the genetic status of the animal gives insight into the expected phenotypes of progeny in the next generation. Even when breeding visually similar animals (eg, black) if the sire is heterozygous and the group of dams he is bred to is heterozygous, then the resulting progeny will be 25% the red coat color. However, if the sire is known to be genetically homozygous for the black coat color, then all progeny will be black, regardless of the genotypic status of the dams.
- Recessive defect detection interrogates the genome for the presence of heritable defects, usually specific for certain breeds, that is, neuropathic hydrocephalus in Angus,[11] cholesterol deficiency,[12] maple syrup urine disease,[13] or mandibulofacial dysostosis[14] in Hereford. Heritable defects are generally recessive, so the presence of the defect is masked in carriers. Defects can be caused by deletions, additions, duplications, or other abnormalities along the genome that might happen during the DNA replication process. Along with parentage testing, determination of the presence of known defects might be required as part of the registration process with the respective breed associations. Defect testing is essential in making informed decisions about breeding pairs.
- Parentage testing verifies the sire and/or dam of a calf. For this type of testing, at least one but ideally both the sire and dam would have genotype profiles available for analysis. Parentage testing is usually based on candidate parents and the analysis is exclusionary in nature.[15] In other words, a relationship between

a calf and a parent is excluded based on the genotyping data, but if a closely related individual to the true parent is considered for evaluation as a parent, it may be accepted as the parent even if the true parent was the closely related individual. Somewhat dependent on genotyping test method (historically STRs, or current state-of-the-art SNPs) and policy of the organization administering the parentage test comparison, a 1% exclusion rate is generally allowed for a calf and one parent relationship, and 1.5% exclusion rate is generally allowed when both parents have the genotype information for parentage analysis.[16]

- Genomic selection evaluates the inheritance of thousands of SNPs across the entire genome to characterize the genetic potential of the animal for many polygenic traits.[17] This process characterizes the mendelian inheritance from parents to offspring earlier in the offspring's life than would be accomplished through own performance recording or progeny performance recording methods. This is an expanded concept from early methods of marker-assisted selection where a few key genetic mutations of biological significance were the basis for selection a few years ago. For additional information, specifically genotyping of dairy cattle, see https://www.ars.usda.gov/ARSUserFiles/80420530/Publications/ARR/Haplotype%20tests_ARR-Genomic5.pdf (accessed 26Apr2024).

Therefore, when a producer indicates they have "genotyped" their animal, it is important to clarify the test that was performed and what the results of that test were. If a client has had an animal parent verified, that is having the animal "genotyped," but it would not provide any insights into the genetic status of that animal for a recessive defect.

Depending on the type of downstream instrumentation used for the final genotyping, some of the preparation for the DNA involves additional pre-steps, adding to the complexity and the time required for completion of tasks. Finally, some of the common methods for genotyping include, but are not limited to, fixed arrays, sequencing (Sanger sequencing or next-generation sequencing), mass spectrometry (MALDI-TOF), and real-time polymerase chain reaction (PCR). It is this instrumentation that then determines the configuration of the genomic DNA, or the genotype. Altogether, laboratory processes are multifaceted and highly complex. Turnaround time of weeks rather than days is an effect of this complexity.

Data Quality Assessment, Data Analysis and Data Interpretation, and Report Generation

The last steps in the process of genotyping start with the verification of data quality. Given that some fixed array platforms return several hundreds of thousands of genotypes per individual animal and sequencing the entire genome returns millions of data points per animal, this process is necessary to verify satisfactory performance of instrumentation and reagents. Depending on the objective of the genotyping, data analysis and data interpretation then generate the report to the client. The report to the client might be an easy to print format with attributes the client will be interested to know about. However, in some cases there may also be more elaborate, interactive, online systems for the client to sort or manipulate the data so that they can utilize the information for their herd management (selection, mating strategies, or even production practices such as generating milk with a specific milk protein profile).

SUMMARY

Outcomes can range from a single "positive/negative" or "favorable/unfavorable" attribute for selection purposes to a complex ranking of animals in a herd by owner-selected traits. Whichever the outcome is, the result is actionable information for the animal owner, helping to make decisions regarding selecting suitable sires and dams to advance improvement goals of herd management, preventing lethal defects from surfacing, identifying the best replacement animals in a herd, and enabling other decisions that impact the likelihood of the owners' success and the well-being of the animals in their care.

CLINICS CARE POINTS

- High-quality sample collection is a fundamental requirement to provide insightful genotyping results to a client.
- Ideal sample collection devices ease the sample collection process on farm, are rapid to deploy on individual animals during routine animal processing, provide a means to store the sample for shipment, and facilitate processing at the genotyping laboratory.
- Knowledge of the genotypic status of animals allows more informed decisions and usage of animals from families which would have historically been avoided because of the risk of unfavorable attributes (eg, carrier of a recessive defect).

ACKNOWLEDGMENTS

The authors gratefully acknowledge the contributions of K.R.L. Cottrell for assistance with figure creation as part of this study.

DISCLOSURE

S. Hinkley and R.G. Tait both work for Neogen Corporation, a commercial genomics service laboratory serving customers in the United States and worldwide.

REFERENCES

1. McGovern SP, Weigel DJ, Fessenden BC, et al. Genomic prediction for twin pregnancies. Animals 2021;11:843–64.
2. Brace MD, Peters O, Menzies P, et al. Sex chromosome chimerism and the freemartin syndrome in Rideau Arcott sheep. Cytogenet Genome Res 2008;120:132–9.
3. Padula AM. The freemartin syndrome: an update. Anim Reprod Sci 2008;87:93–109.
4. Hykin SM, Bi K, McGuire JA. Fixing Formalin: A method to recover genomic-scale DNA sequence data from formalin-fixed museum specimens using high-throughput sequencing. PLoS One 2015;10(10):e0141579. https://doi.org/10.1371/journal.pone.0141579.
5. Dechow CD, Frye E, Maunsell FP. Identification of a putative haplotype associated with recumbency in Holstein calves. JDS Comms 2022;3:412–5.
6. Brooks JW. Postmortem changes in animal carcasses and estimation of the postmortem interval. Vet Pathol 2016;52:929–40.
7. Almulhim AM, Menezes RG. Evaluation of postmortem changes. In: StatPearls. Treasure Island (FL): StatPearls Publishing; 2024. Available at: https://www.ncbi.nlm.nih.gov/books/NBK554464/.
8. Heyen DW, Beever JE, Da Y, et al. Exclusion probabilities of 22 bovine microsatellite markers in fluorescent multiplexes for semi-automated parentage testing. Anim Genet 1997;28:21–7.

9. MacHugh DE, Loftus RT, Cunningham P, et al. Genetic structure of seven European cattle breeds assessed using 20 microsatellite markers. Anim Genet 1998;29:333–40.

10. Matukumalli LK, Lawley CT, Schnabel RD, et al. Development and characterization of a high density SNP genotyping assay for cattle. PLoS One 2009;4(4): e5350. https://doi.org/10.1371/journal.pone.0005350.

11. Available at: https://www.angus.org/Pub/NH/NHInfo. [Accessed 26 April 2024].

12. Menzi F, Besuchet-Schmutz N, Fragnière M, et al. A transposable element insertion in *APOB* causes cholesterol deficiency in Holstein cattle. Anim Genet 2016; 47:253–7.

13. Zhang B, Healy PJ, Zhao Y, et al. Premature translation termination of the pre-E1α subunit of the branched chain α–ketoacid dehydrogenase as a cause of Maple Syrup Urine Disease in polled Hereford calves. J Biol Chem 1990;265:2425–7.

14. Sieck RL, Fuller AM, Bedwell RP, et al. Mandibulofacial Dysostosis attributed to a recessive mutation of *CYP26C1* in Hereford cattle. Genes 2020;11:1246–58.

15. Jamieson A, Taylor ST. Comparisons of three probability formulae for parentage exclusion. Anim Genet 1997;28:397–400.

16. Meuwissen THE, Hayes BJ, Goddard ME. Prediction of total genetic value using genomie-wide dense marker maps. Genetics 2001;157:1819–29.

17. International Council on Animal Recording. ICAR guidelines for parentage verification and parentage discovery based on SNP genotypes. 2017. Available at: https://www.icar.org/Documents/GenoEx/ICAR%20Guidelines%20for%20Parentage%20Verification%20and%20Parentage%20Discovery%20based%20on%20SNP.pdf.

The Private Practitioner

A Veterinary Practitioner's Perspective to the Application of Bovine Genomics in Client Herds

Patrick M.R. Comyn, DVM

KEYWORDS

• Genomics • Genetics • Epigenomics • Generation interval

KEY POINTS

- Genomic evaluation has changed how sires are selected in the major dairy and beef breeds.
- The rate of genetic progress in some breeds of cattle has accelerated with genomics.
- Genomic evaluation allows breeders to directly select traits that one cannot visualize.
- Genomic evaluation reveals an accurate genetic evaluation at a very young age.

Genomic evaluation, based on the Illumina chip where between 3000 and 700,000 single nucleotide polymorphisms (SNPs) are evaluated, has had profound effects on the dairy and beef industry globally.[1] When incorporated into preexisting production metrics, genomic testing data increase the reliability of trait measurements.

The probability of identifying a positive trait increases with improved trait reliability. Veterinarians need to be aware of the impact genomic testing can have on animal health and productivity. Genomic Predicted Transmitting Abilities (PTAs) and Expected Progeny Differences (EPDs) can be utilized in dairy and beef breeding respectively to assess udder health, docility, propensity to remain on the farm, reproductive performance, carcass characteristics, and so forth. In the future, more in-depth genome analysis involving a manyfold increase in SNP will allow for the evaluation and selection of traits such as susceptibility to respiratory disease, parasitism, and other pathologic conditions.

Since 2009, the Holstein and Jersey breeds (the primary dairy breed participants percentage wise in genomic testing) have witnessed a 192% increase in productive traits, largely due to greater and less biased young sire screening for admission to progeny testing and decreased generational time.[2]

Virginia Herd Health Management Service P.C, PO Box 555, Madison, VA 22727, USA
E-mail address: pcomyn@verizon.net

Vet Clin Food Anim 40 (2024) 399–413
https://doi.org/10.1016/j.cvfa.2024.05.005
vetfood.theclinics.com

INTRODUCTION

As a veterinarian who has practiced bovine medicine throughout his entire career, this article is intended to address the role of a private veterinary practitioner in the utilization of genomic predictions to assist dairy and beef clients. I became involved in bovine genomics as an extension of my business in embryo transfer, which involved the sale and export of embryos and live cattle from Holsteins and Angus cattle to Japan, Russia, the European Union, Uruguay, China, and Australia. Utilizing genomic preexisting production metrics was a natural extension of the business I was involved with. I have had no formal training in molecular or population genetics. My education has come from many thousands of dollars spent on genomic testing cattle I have owned and then discussing the results, and the bigger picture thereof, with those that I regarded and still regard as experts in the art and science of breeding cattle. Those people include bull stud sire selection personnel, livestock sale agents, geneticists, dairy and beef producers, university personnel, and a few veterinarians. They are the people that anyone interested in gaining knowledge about bovine genomics, genetics, and epigenetics should become acquainted with.

Genomic genetic evaluation has been one of the most transformative technologies in animal agriculture since artificial insemination became widely used in the 1950s following the development of techniques to freeze and then successfully thaw semen. The fundamentals of healthier, more efficient cattle in an economically resilient dairy or beef operation lies, in part, in constant development and utilization of reliable genetic trait prediction. Genetic alignment determines the limits of trait expression; management or animal husbandry plus genetic alignment determines measurable trait expression.[3] How do we develop a role for the practitioner in on-farm genetic management? A good place to start is to understand the origins of dairy genetics.

At its heart, genetics is a study of recorded measurements of phenotypes, which reflect phenotypic variation. To accurately prove that a male or female is truly superior to herd mates, genetically contemporary, or related individuals at separate locations requires a lot of records with consistent phenotypic reporting. The Local Dairy Herd Improvement Associations (DHIA) and national dairy breed associations have been collecting cow production and type data for over 100 years.[4] The United States Department of Agriculture Animal Improvement Program Laboratory (USDA-AIPL), animal geneticists at United States land-grant universities, and similar institutions outside of the United States have made formulas using these data to yield PTA metrics (similar to EPD in the US beef industry) for dairy animals and broader-based multi-trait PTA indices such as Net Merit indices from the USDA and later the Council for Dairy Cattle Breeding (CDCB)[5] and Type Production Indices (TPI) from dairy breed associations. TPI from dairy breed associations brings more emphasis on the physical appearance of a cow as is recorded by dairy classifiers at type classification than does USDA/CDCB lifetime Net Merit or similar indices.

Net Merit, TPI, and similar metrics utilize trait PTAs proportionately in the stated index. The proportion to which a production index utilizes an individual metric such as productive life (PL) or protein production (PRO) reflects the percentage, on average, that this metric contributes to the measured productive value of an animal against an average herd mate. In the figure below (**Fig. 1**) showing trait contribution in the 2021 lifetime Net Merit formula, PL is 15% of the total net merit value.

Prior to genomic evaluation, the lifetime Net Merit metric was not calculated by the USDA-AIPL until the animal had largely completed her first lactation. The generational interval in dairy breeds was about 7 years. The genetic value of a dairy female was not known until she was two and a half to 4 years old. At present, one can genomically test

Weighting of Traits in Net Merit Dollars ($)

Holstein

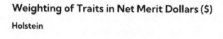
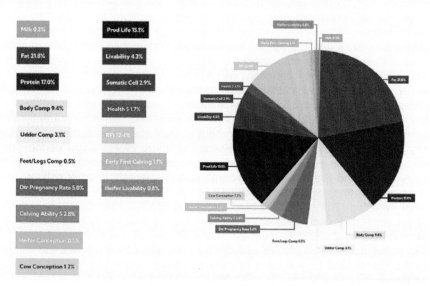

Milk 0.3%	Prod Life 15.1%
Fat 21.8%	Livability 4.3%
Protein 17.0%	Somatic Cell 2.9%
Body Comp 9.4%	Health $ 1.7%
Udder Comp 3.1%	RFI 12.4%
Feet/Legs Comp 0.5%	Early First Calving 1.1%
Dtr Pregnancy Rate 5.0%	Heifer Livability 0.8%
Calving Ability $ 2.8%	
Heifer Conception 0.5%	
Cow Conception 1.2%	

Fig. 1. CDCB Net Merit Formula 2021 trait PTA contributions. (CDCB, August 2021- https://uscdcb.com/wp-content/uploads/2021/06/NM-2021-Frequent-Questions-06_07_2021.pdf.)

a young heifer and within a few weeks have in hand as much or more genetic information on this calf as a sixth or seventh lactation cow might have had before genomic testing. A very important point to consider is that genomic evaluation in cattle and incorporation into pre-existing production metrics is only valuable in the breeds with large numbers of production records. In the USA dairy industry, genomics currently has the greatest impact on Holsteins and Jerseys. For beef breeds, Angus, Red Angus, and Simmental possess the greatest record base for developing predictions. The smaller breeds can be tested, however, the progeny equivalents added to their PTAs or EPDs by genomic testing are far less than the larger breeds mentioned. On a similar note, it must be acknowledged that advances seen in the production of dairy cattle in the United States are largely attributable to production data given voluntarily and without remuneration, by producers to the DHIA and thence breed organizations and the USDA-AIPL. Since animal genomes can change quite rapidly from generation to generation, current genomic patterns today lose accuracy with each succeeding generation, unless the genomic "bank" is updated routinely with production data from the current generation. We can call this "genetic drift" or the point of the spear of evolution. A practitioner can be instrumental in encouraging clients to submit production data to breed and management (DHI) associations. Individual animal data submission is vital for accurate production metrics for each breed. It is also important to note that a genotype/phenotype relationship in one breed (breed A), does not necessarily translate to another (breed B). The variation in genetic patterns is breed specific.

Dairy genetic advancement began with the establishment of breed associations and dairy herd improvement associations in the late 19th and early 20th centuries.

The dairy industry developed and utilized metrics devised by the USDA-AIPL, State Land Grant University scientists, scientists in agricultural universities in countries other than the USA, the USA and foreign breed associations, and later (in the United States) the CDCB in the attempt to breed a better cow. The theme in dairy breeding up until the 1970s and early 80s could be summed up as "form to function" by which if you breed them to look like dairy cattle and manage them like dairy cattle, they will perform like dairy cattle. Dairy cattle evaluation (judging) was an important part of this selection method as was the collection of production data such as milk yield and fat, then protein percentages. Many traits which presently are found to be very important from a management perspective, such as reproductive indices and milk quality indices, were not included in early estimations of value. Economic conditions on dairy farms in the USA became more rigorous post-1945, while concurrently consumer demand for higher quality milk products (shelf life, flavor, texture) grew. The dairy (and beef) industry needed to develop metrics to evaluate cow performance and bull trait transmission. These metrics developed by or in conjunction with the USDA, State Land Grant University scientists, and scientists in other nations, predicted genetic transmission to offspring and were dubbed PTA in dairy and Estimated Breeding Value or EPD in beef. Reproduction and udder health were found to have some degree of heritability and thus were eventually included in genetic appraisals done by the USDA, Land Grant Universities, and similar organizations in other countries. A limiting factor in these trait prediction formulas was the number of offspring required to give proof to a measurement. A cow had too few offspring and lactations in her lifetime to draw many conclusions about her genetic value. Thus, most of a cow's genetic value was derived from her sire stack data. A bull usually has many more offspring to develop an idea of his genetic value. This is especially true of a bull used for artificial insemination utilizing fresh or frozen semen. Therefore, traditionally the genetic value of a dairy female was largely derived from the performance of the sires in her pedigree, (with large numbers of offspring in many herds), with some of her own individual performance being factored in as that data became available. That cow's production data were judged against other half-siblings and closely related peers to assess if she outperformed, underperformed, or was equal to her peers. All things considered, a female dairy cow (or beef cow, for that matter) had a relatively low reliability to her genetic valuation prior to genomic testing. Another, less complicated way to express this is that the range of possible variation from that animal's calculated PTAs or EPDs was quite large. This was also true with bulls pre-genomically, but bulls will increase reliability rapidly once daughters come into production—especially if the daughters were in different herds under different management and environments.

Base Changes

This brings us to the question of "how do genetic evaluations remain current to the population being assessed?" In the dairy breed genetic sector, initially the USDA-AIPL and now the US-CDCB does what is called a base change once every 5 years. Performance data from all dairy animals in the queried base year (current base year in 2024 is 2015) are utilized to evaluate and standardize the data of animals moving forward the next 5 years. When a base change occurs, PTA metrics on essentially all evaluated cattle are pulled back toward the base mean as the "average" Holstein female born in 2015 will have a $NM (dollar US Net Merit) of 0 (zero). Therefore if she was born in 2019 and tested genomically in 2019 (being too young to have meaningful performance data), the genomic metrics would have been evaluated through the lens of the 2010 base or the average cow in 2010. Her PTAs would probably be superior to the base in 2010 (or maybe not). When base change occurred in 2020, the heifer's PTAs would be pulled back in equal measure to the broader base change to that of an average cow born in 2015. At current genetic improvement pace, sire intergenerational interval is less than 3 years so the sire stack on this heifer could move by 1.5 to 2 generations. It is worth noting that all the metrics change due to the populational trait movements. But change on each sire is a culmination of new daughter data. This way comparison of animals across age and genetic ranges is possible. Base change prevents genetic inflation.[6,7]

Dairy producers and beef producers have had (and still have) differing ideas on what made for a "better" cow. Some producers have desired cows that scored well in breed classification programs, feeling that the structural traits in high-scoring cows enable these cows to have increased performance and longevity. These producers had been taught through 4-H, FFA, judging teams, etc. that a visible physical trait such as a wide spring of ribs, might also confer traits such as longer PL or more milk production via greater capacity for feed intake. These producers were attempting to link unseen or difficult-to-see traits, (positively or negatively), by increasing or decreasing traits easily seen and easily measured. The idea that a "competent" cattle person can "see" a superior animal is still utilized post-genomically in dairy cattle but is much more prevalent in the beef world, where a good or bad photograph can have a substantial impact on sales of bull semen. Now that genomic testing is widely available, many producers (beef and dairy) utilize more production-based metrics to directly address characteristics that are not visible, such as daughter pregnancy rate or PL. Rather than using breed PTAs on moderately to highly heritable phenotypic traits such as height and udder suspension to hopefully link to unseen traits; producers consistently utilizing direct measurement of a trait can move the herd in a desired direction more rapidly and consistently than one attempting to gain access to a trait via hoped for linkage with a more visible trait. An example would be using bulls with low somatic cell score (SCS) PTA to support a genetic basis for the low SCS, as opposed to selecting a bull with a PTA of 4 standard deviations above the group mean for udder composite to achieve a low SCS. A high udder composite PTA will yield offspring udders that are well above the tarsus and that have a well-defined median support ligament. By selecting for teats that are less likely to become covered with bacteria from manure (not close to the ground) and making udders that are more conducive to milking unit placement and function, the cow with these traits will tend to have less udder health issues compared to a cow with a pendulous udder. These producers, who utilized a direct trait metric, such as SCS PTA selected for this trait without depending on selection for a secondary trait that might or might not have an association with the primary (desired) trait—that is, not all bulls that have a high (visually desirable to a dairy person) udder comp PTA have a correspondingly low SCA PTA. Many producers now use some portions of type assessment and some direct trait selection. A producer might want all bulls to have an udder composite PTA greater than 1 standard deviation and an SCS PTA less than let us say 2.8.

Some trait PTAs that one cannot easily "see" visually.
These include.

- Productive life
- Livability
- Health traits
- Future conception rate differential from peers of her daughters
- Her conception rate differential from peers
- Feed efficiency

DISCUSSION

Prior to the advent of genomics, many commercial dairy producers and dairy production-oriented veterinarians believed that genetic advancement/management was of minor importance; they felt that environmental management advancement was paramount—if one fed a consistent, properly formulated ration and kept the cows in a clean, dry, comfortable environment, the cows would perform in an acceptable manner regardless of genetics. This point of view, to me, was a back door admission, to the slow pace and imprecise movement of dairy genetic generational improvement. Similarly, the slow pace of genetic improvement/lack of EPD reliability in beef cattle also accounts in part for beef producers using crossbreeding (heterosis) to bring in favorable traits as opposed to same-breed bull selection on single-breed/purebred cows.

Veterinarians traditionally have not spent much time in genetic management, in part because that industry space was occupied by bull studs and university extension services and because our formal training does not allow much—if any time to this area. A lot of veterinary practitioners seem to regard genetic expression as a binary, yes or no, proposition. An example of this is having horns—a highly heritable trait where homozygous x homozygous horns = horns, heterozygous x heterozygous = 25% horns (homozygous), 50% polled (heterozygous–carriers) and 25% polled (homozygous polled). The reality of genetics is that most traits we value have heritability of 1% to around 40%, with many traits being in the 10% to 20% heritability range. This means that the environment (management) is responsible for the majority of trait expression. A trait such as milk fat yield or adult height might have a heritability of say 40%. Management (Environment) then is responsible for 60% of the trait expression. Intervention on highly heritable traits can lead to rapid gains in genetic progress, but this does not preclude selection for low heritability traits being useful. Like compounded interest, ignoring these traits adds up and can have large impacts. This was seen in Holstein's reproductive performance from the 1980s up until about 2010.[8] Another concept to keep in mind is reliability. Reliability is the accuracy of the trait measurement or better said, the range of possible outcomes for that trait in an individual. An example is birth weight (BW). If a bull or cow has a PTA or EPD showing a BW (Birth Weight) of −0.5 lb. with reliability of that metric of 05 or 5%; the range of possible outcomes at that reliability will be large perhaps or exceeding −3 lb. to +4 lb. with any point in that range being equally possible. The true BW, once enough offspring are generated to provide statistical proof, might end up being +3 lb. at 70% reliability and maybe +2.25 lb. at 99% reliability off of the original prediction (and that movement can be either greater or less than the original prediction). The author feels that many practitioners have seen this with frustrated clients stating that "the bull is supposed to be calving ease'and then be shown the registration papers showing that prediction. Pre-genomic testing, genetic progress was a slow-moving business with a bull taking 6 or 7 years from birth until enough daughters had completed a first lactation to achieve reliable proof.[9] It was often said by dairy genetics professors that the best bulls in the Holstein population each year were harvested as veal due to the inability at that time to identify superior genetics (due to an inability to sample but so many bulls a year both in facilities and cost both to purchase and maintain more bulls). In addition to lacking facilities and money to more bulls, the bull stud sire procurement departments really did not know where to look for young herd sire prospects except through known cow families.

As Sattler wrote in 2013, in 2004 to 2008 about 1200 dairy bulls were in progeny testing at any time in North American bull studs. Post-genomically the number of bulls evaluated annually (with most not being selected) grew into the tens of thousands (including genomic tested and rejected and those genomically tested and accepted).

The actual number of bulls purchased for progeny testing (all dairy bulls purchased in the United States and Canada by bull studs that are able to successfully freeze semen will be in progeny testing) decreased post genomically.[10] Pre-genomically bulls that were purchased as young sires (consideration for sire status was based on parent-average PTA, pedigree, and cow family promotion by owners) failed to be proven superior and thus were culled. A small number of bulls emerged each year as new proven sires. It is worth noting that prior to around 2005, there really were not many performance measurements available to consider. Milk production, fat, protein, somatic cell, sire conception rate, type metrics, and sire stack (sire stack being the paternal lineage of an individual) were the main considerations. Most bull studs had mating services that would match up cows in a herd to that bull stud's lineup based on owner trait preferences.

A large element of unknown in sire proofing existed because of the level of misidentification that occurred on calf identity.[11] This was often not realized until the "second crop" of calves came into lactation some 3 to 4 years after the bull's small initial (proofing) release. A calf sired by an unproven young sire would have the PTA reliability (based on parent average PTA) of approximately 15% or so which is the cow genetic equivalent of perhaps 2 to 4 offspring having completed a lactation. A calf sired by a proven sire stack might have a reliability of 35% to 38%, which would add several more cow equivalents to the calf's proof. Now with genomic evaluation, a genomic-tested Holstein calf's genomic prediction reliability will be from around 60% to over 80%, depending on trait. Overall reliability on genomic prediction will be over 70%.[12]

Dairy-oriented veterinary practice since the mid-1990s has been defined by change at a rate not experienced in the past. Among these changes are geographic relocation of dairy production areas, integration and expansion of information technologies, handheld computing, gender-selected semen, and genomic prediction of genetic trait transmitting ability. So, the question being posed is "where does the veterinarian on a farm fit into the use and analysis of genetic trait transmission?" Do veterinarians have a role in the use of genomic information on the farm?

I am going to say "Yes; the practitioner does have a role." To quote Fred Gingrich, DVM, current director of the American Association of Bovine Practitioners, "We (veterinarians) should be the cow's advocate." But to address the question, I will address what, in this practitioner's view, genomic evaluation brings to animal health and productivity that should be of interest to us.

The "what" genomic evaluation offers from a veterinary practitioners perspective is 4-fold

A. Timeliness. Help manage the replacement pool size at an early age.
B. Ability to measure economically important traits and use them in breeding management.
   a. Trait selection criteria in sire pool to match female trait selection with female gender selected dairy on dairy breeding.
C. Ranking of lactating females to make breeding decisions.
   a. Beef on dairy or dairy on dairy.
      i. Gender-sorted (dairy or beef) or conventional semen (dairy or beef).
D. A genomic-tested heifer has the same genetic impact or weight as a genomic-tested bull—embryo transfer or genetic sale potential.

To highlight the importance of timeliness, consider that prior to genomic-enhanced PTAs, developing a highly reliable PTA proof on a dairy bull took 8 to 10 years. Because of errors in animal ID and breeding recordings, among others, the accuracy of a bull's initial proof was often less accurate than it appeared. Traditionally, it took another large round of offspring (formerly called the second proof) for the PTAs on a bull to stabilize. Prior to Illumina-chip-based genomic testing, the decision on which Holstein bull calf to select from a group resulting from an embryo transfer procedure was arbitrary. This was because all of the young calves from a flush had identical parent average PTAs. Of a group of say 2 to 6 male flush mates, no one knew which bull calf was the best, worst, or average. Now, using genomic predictions, the Holstein calves can be ranked before weaning with the analytical strength equivalent to 100+ calves in its genomic proof. The strongest point of comparison in genomics is between full siblings.

TRAIT ASSESSMENT

One can observe certain traits like stature, milk production, and udder composite with a minimum of training and use these observations to make breeding decisions. This approach has been the backbone of dairy breeding since its inception as a science 100+ years ago. However, there are important traits that cannot be seen *in situ* and therefore are considered prospective. Here is an incomplete list of these.

- Productive life
- Livability
- Gestation length
- Daughter pregnancy rate
- Feed efficiency

These traits are quantified in a metric via genomic testing and incorporation into PTAs. If one can identify and measure a trait, one can plan how to or if to select for and/or manage this trait.

UTILIZATION OF TRAIT PREDICTION IN A BREEDING PROGRAM

These trait prediction metrics are important contributors to composite tools such as $ lifetime net merit, dairy wellness profit $, TPI, LPI (Lifetime Profit Index - a Canadian index), and other composite tools that are used by dairy producers to assess the potential monetary value that a heifer might bring to the herd, or the real monetary value that a cow brings to the herd compared, to that animal's peers. The formulae are adjusted at a set schedule (in the United States, for dairy animals, every 5 years by the US-CDCB) to reflect the real-world cost of production, product value, and genetic currentness of the population of peers. This way the formula remains relevant for comparison. These unseen traits comprise about 47% of the Lifetime Net Merit formula in US dairy cows. If one counts an accurate measure of milk solids yield on a non-lactating heifer, the "unseen" portion of genomic testing on $NM and other similar formulae increase dramatically. Net Merit and other like indices in the US dairy industry are applied to all commercial dairy breeds and to dairy x dairy crossbred cattle if the animal is in a herd enrolled in the DHIA or a similar testing method where animal data go back to the CDCB.

The practitioner involved with genetic decisions should consider that management can provide an environment so that a trait is to be expressed to its fullest extent. But the DNA of the subject controls what that extent might be. Therefore, by employing genomically enhanced PTAs (or EPDs) one can set parameters for genetic advancement using Holstein or Jersey young sires (1 to one and a half years old) with confidence that within a group, the group average would move in a desired fashion.

The genomically tested female carries as much genetic prescience or value as a genomically tested male without offspring. This is not really a change from pre-genomic valuations except that the metrics involved have much greater reliability and so less room for significant movement of a metric as more data are added to the production proof.

A genomically tested female carries the same progeny equivalents as a genomically tested (but not daughter-proven) male, enabling a more straightforward path of genetic advancement with significantly fewer detours than was achievable prior to genomically enhanced PTA/EPDs. Original estimates in Holstein cattle for increases in daughter equivalents by genomically tested females over traditional proofing, at the advent of genomic testing in 2008, was around 15 to 20 progeny equivalent lactating daughters, but with the large increase in genomic tested Holsteins (over 8 million head), the number of daughter equivalents has grown substantially.[13,14] This situation has never existed before in cattle breeding. The exploitation of this development is why there has been a huge increase in advanced reproductive techniques (Embryo transfer both in-vivo and in-vitro) utilized in young dairy heifers in the past 10 years or so.

Most projects on a dairy operation undertaken to improve cow or heifer productivity and health require time, money, space, and extensive planning to bring the improvements to bear. Genetic advancement, however, differs slightly in its approach; it requires the insemination of a female bovine for her to become pregnant, give birth, and commence a new. The question then becomes "Do we want more of an individual cow's genetics in the herd?" With the yes option, there are several points to consider.

1. Build a list of acceptable sires realizing that there is no perfect bull or perfect mating.
2. Keep trait selection simple, select 3 or 4 traits or metrics that are important.
   a. Realize that heritability matters in terms of trait impact.
      i. Heritability + environment = trait expression.
      ii. It is wise, in my opinion, to first consider a multi-trait production index such as Net Merit, LPI (Canada), TPI, $C (Angus), API Simmental.
1. Use a broad index for the initial sire cut.
2. If using cow phenotype evaluation (classification or evaluation) then one can make pools of cows whose offspring might need longer teats, better foot angle, higher fat percentage, and so forth.
   a. Then make a sub list of bulls that accomplish what is desired.

I think in breeding commercial dairy cattle, it is important not to get into too much detail on sire selection. Find a set of sires that accomplish most of the desired criteria, then move on to other tasks. Using broad indices accomplishes this. No bull is perfect.

The other side of genomic usage in dairy cattle has been the use of beef sires on dairy females with lower-ranking genetic merit. Several technologies arrived in the cattle reproduction world in close order to each other and complemented each other.

1. Sex-selected semen.
2. Genomic testing.
3. Improved calf care/calf survivability.
4. Recognizing and managing periparturient nutritional requirements to decrease postpartum metabolic disease incidence.

Raising replacement heifers is both expensive and resource intensive. The use of gender-selected semen, genomic evaluation, and better overall management resulting in lower cull rates has allowed producers to target the females that they do not wish to have replacement females from. An example of the 4 points was a conversation I had with Gordie Jones, DVM in 2020 where the Wisconsin dairy operation, where he was a managing partner, had an involuntary (deaths, reproductive culls, chronic mastitis, chronic foot problem) cull rate of about 13% to 15%. This gives a tremendous opportunity to cut back on a large expenditure—namely, that of raising heifers. Cows still need to become pregnant to initiate a new lactation. The solution to needing less dairy replacement heifers is to use beef semen to inseminate cows whose genetics are not desired. The cattle industry calls these calves "Beef on Dairy." The beef x dairy cross calves generally bring a greater return to the farm than a pure dairy bull calf. When one jumps from the dairy side of the bovine world to the beef side, one jumps into a different vocabulary regarding production metrics. The beef associations have developed what they call EPD in place of the PTA. The 2 terms basically mean the same thing. It is important to recognize that dairy PTAs usually utilize standard deviation from a group statistical mean to describe differences between individuals; beef EPDs utilize percentile ranking within the breed to describe differences. Beef organizations do not have cross beef breeds standardized set of EPD metrics or standardized index EPDs such as the dairy industry does. There are interbreed data models to predict some of the trait outcomes of crossbreeding in beef herds when crossing breed A to breed B utilizing the breed EPDs for each breed.[9]

At present (2023–2024) in the beef-on-dairy semen market, the Angus breed accounts for more than 88% of semen straws sold to dairy operations. Some of the beef breed associations, using genomic evaluation, rank-tested males for their suitability on dairy breeds. This information can be found by going to the appropriate breed association website and entering a bull's registered name or registration number in the EPD look-up. Bull studs also list some beef bulls that they market for applicability to the beef on the dairy market. The beef-on-dairy transition is not driven by science and research projects. Rather it is an innovative market-driven approach that, in the author's discussions with industry people, is a phenomenon that research is struggling to address and catch up with. This market is driven by economic and biological realities on the dairy side—the need to get dairy cows pregnant to calve and thus lactate and the greater value in a beef-on-dairy calf than on a dairy calf destined for slaughter. The beef-on-dairy strategy has had a profound effect on the beef bull market for those beef seedstock producers that sell bulls to bull studs or in some cases directly to large dairy producers. In the latter case, the bulls are going to private semen collection centers and the dairy operations are having the bull semen collected and frozen for on-farm use. The notable impact on the bull seedstock market is attributable to the US beef cow herd, which numbers approximately 29 million head.[15] Of these, maybe 11% to 12% of operations utilize AI in their breeding management.[16] The USDA 2017 NAHMS report highlighted about 95% of mature beef cow groups were bred solely to bulls and about 89% of heifers were bred solely to bulls.[16] The US dairy herd is about 9 million head,[17] but a very large percentage of the cows and heifers within the dairy sector will be bred by artificial insemination and multiple times at that.[18] From 2017 through 2021 beef semen sales rose by 260% while dairy semen sales dropped by 24%.[19,20] Some of the bull studs offer dairy producers a shortened set of metrics in beef on dairy bulls where calving data, weaning/yearling weight (YW) and carcass merit are emphasized. This is reasonable as these calves are destined for slaughter, not breeding. Interestingly, the beef breed associations stand to benefit from beef on dairy since these result in identified and genomically tested calves that can be tracked through feeding and slaughter. Carcass data, feed-out data, and health performance data can be collected and go to breed associations allowing for enhanced genomic predictions for the sire and the dam's sire stack. Over time the author feels that carcass merit will be included in Holstein and Jersey genomic predictions, as the beef on dairy calves will gain favor and value in the beef market, due to consumers favoring the consistency of the beef on dairy meat products.

Characteristics being evaluated in beef sires being used to produce semen for beef on dairy.

- Calving ease
- Sold calf weight at a week or so of age
- Weaning weight
- Yearling weight
- Height
- Carcass weight
- Carcass yield
- Ribeye area
- Size of cut
- Marbling
- Grade
- Consumer approval of product cut appearance on a grocery store shelf.

I believe that rather than trying to breed for those individual traits, one can get more done by using a breed association-generated index such as the $AxH from the American Angus Association; the following description is copied with permission from the American Angus Association 2023.[21]

Angus – On - Holstein ($AxH), a terminal index, expressed in dollars per head, to predict profitability differences in progeny due to genetic traits weighted by appropriated economics of each Angus sire when mated to Holstein females. The underlying breeding objective assumes Angus bulls will be mated to Holstein females to produce Angus-dairy crossbred calves to be fed and marketed on a quality-based grid. Traits included are as follows: calving ease, growth from birth through the feeding phase, feed intake, dressing percent, yield grade, quality grade, muscling, and height.

The $AxH index will indicate a specific Angus sire's ranking against other contemporary Angus sires, where 1% is very desirable and 95% is quite a bit less desirable. It is the author's opinion that when using beef on dairy in mature dairy cows or heifers one should look at Calving Ease Direct (CED) and BW to get an indication of anticipated ease of calving, especially if using gender-sorted male semen. Crossbred calves tend to be heavier than purebred calves by a kilogram or 2 and bull calves tend to weigh more than heifer calves.[22,23]

The purpose of beef on dairy is firstly, to enable a successful lactation, and secondly, to market a beef cross calf that has more value than what a dairy bull calf might be worth. Dystocia can affect both of those objectives. The use of genomics in bulls from beef breeds with more production data, allows us to identify potential sires that have a high CED (meaning easy calving), low BW (lower BW calves tend to be born easier), and yet have a high Weaning Weight and YW, reflecting growth potential. How this might get utilized depends on the dairy operation's method of calf marketing—meaning, does the dairy operation management wish for a relationship with a feeder/packer where carcass quality, yield, efficiency, and sire identity are prioritized, or is the beef calf to be sold simply as a beef calf with no identity attached. It has been expressed to the author by multiple AI Sire procurement personnel, that there is no real plan in the beef on dairy usage. It is sort of cut and fit or changed on a day-to-day or week-to-week basis. Numerous metrics play a role in the use of beef on dairy genetics, a few of these being in importance per bull stud representatives.

1. Sire conception rate
2. Availability of gender-selected semen (male being preferred)
3. Weight of beef x dairy calf sold (>38 Kg is highly desirable)
4. Dystocia incidence
5. Carcass characteristics

It is worth noting that an operation that does not retain a financial interest in the calf's post-sale might be more interested in points 1 to 3 whereas an operation that retains some financial interest in the calves through slaughter might have a different weighting on sire selection importance. Again, since beef on dairy is a recent, market-driven, phenomenon, there is not much in the way of studies to reference.

The $AxH or $AxJ index gives an estimate of the final terminal value of a calf sired by bull N x Average Holstein or Jersey dam versus one sired by an average Angus bull. This index is looked at in $ and in percentage against the breed. Jersey producers seem to be using more Continental-type breeds such as Simmental or Limousin as they add more carcass weight than perhaps Angus does whereas Holstein producers are utilizing more of smaller stature angus to yield offspring with desired slaughter characteristics. The bull studs are developing market entry/market access tools to connect dairy producers selling calves sired by high terminal value sires to feedyards. The calves involved in these transactions are generally managed according to a protocol of colostrum management, measured serum total protein, vaccines, and so forth.

The AI industry is also developing hybrid lines with multiple sire lines being used in dairy crosses. The difficulty that I see with this approach is in the increased potential for variation in outcomes due to the genetic diversity when one crosses, say, a 4-way hybrid to a Holstein or Jersey. The genetic stability of such a cross would, to me, come more from the dairy side than the beef cross, except that the desired traits from the dairy side are not measured in a PTA or EPD in dairy genetic testing. In the end, the market will give guidance as to what is the most desirable cross with beef on dairy. That market decision will be a combination of total feedlot/slaughter performance and consumer-driven acceptance of the beef products—taste x texture x appearance x price.

Epigenetics—where the genome meets the environment and becomes a bovine.

Epigenetics, as it impacts animal appearance and performance, starts as a riddle and ends up as the animal that we see. I regard epigenetic gene expression as the big unknown in dairy (and beef) genetic evaluation. In a nutshell, genetic transfer is the result of spermatid/oocyte production, meiosis, fertilization, formation of a zygote, then an embryo, then a fetus, and finally a live calf. At points of spermatid/oocyte development, zygote/embryo development, fetal development, and then birth and beyond, DNA segments are activated or deactivated via the addition or removal of methyl or acetyl groups. This is partly driven by environmental conditions that the dam, sire, and conceptus experience on a day-to-day basis—environmental adaptation. This concept is perhaps the most important piece of the genetic puzzle and yet the most difficult part to predict from one genotype to another. It is old wisdom that some well-managed herd has "good, dependable" cattle, yet this wisdom is true. We know that farm management plays a huge role in epigenetic expression by managing feed quality and quantity, heat abatement, cow comfort, air quality, animal stress/anxiety, and so forth.[24] This is true in other species as well including humans.[25]

As a veterinarian and the cow's advocate, one must realize that stress/unfavorable situations involving cattle that reproduce, (male and female), will have consequences somewhere in the future in the current generation, the next, or even subsequent generations. Stress-free livestock production is important; a veterinary practitioner should endeavor to work to alleviate bottlenecks in a production unit, using the knowledge that production bottlenecks equal stress, and stress equals unfavorable epigenetic effects. The ultimate arbiter of our animal care decisions and efforts, the consumer, does and will demand no less. Unfavorable, management-related epigenetic effects are expensive to correct if they can be corrected at all.

SUMMARY

This article aims to persuade fellow practitioners to look at the technology of genomics not as a new phenomenon but rather as an extension of tools we have been using in bovine management for the last 40 years or so. As with many measurements frequently used, the accuracy of the measurement improves over time due to technological changes and the accumulation of data. Genomics and data management have also allowed for new metrics, important to dairy and beef production, to be recognized and utilized. Phenotypic data are at the heart of genomic technology. Tomorrow's genomic predictions are only valid if present-time phenotypic data are made available to breed associations, industry data management associations, and the USDA, or like organizations to factor genetic drift over time. Breeding philosophy is important—what traits are important and how should one rank them? For this, I can only advise keeping the system of selection simple, choose 3 or 4 traits to emphasize and leave the rest alone. If one tries to bring in too many traits, one will end up with no bulls in the selected group. As previously mentioned, I use a major index as my first selector, look over this group and then decide how much harder to cut. Remember—no bull is perfect. Genomic analysis which examines 10,000 to 50,000 SNPs has begun a revolution in animal selection and has allowed us to evaluate production traits that we heretofore have not been able to "see." New methods of genome evaluation, capable of reading tens to hundreds of times more SNPs on the genome, such as Low Pass Whole Genome Sequencing are on the horizon. These new technologies, coupled with phenotypic data hold the potential to solve questions that we have been struggling with, such as susceptibility to disease, reproductive loss, heat intolerance, and so forth. A practitioner must understand that one does not have to understand all points of genomic analysis, to see the importance of a basic understanding of genomics in an agricultural system.

CLINICS CARE POINTS

Genomic evaluation of dairy cattle, when integrated with existing PTA, is a relatively new look at an existing and evolving technology. Some questions that can assist the practitioner in guiding a client with genomic technology include.

- What sorts of traits does one want to concentrate on with dairy-on-dairy genetics?
- If using beef on dairy, what is important to the client—calf price, dairy replacement value and availability, calving ease, conception rate, and cost of semen?
- Regarding beef on dairy, is the client aware of industry data showing the profitability of crosses of a dairy breed or a dairy breed blend (Holstein/Jersey) by different beef breeds or beef hybrids?
- Is there reliable data showing the net impact of beef on dairy breeding where the calf size increases (especially bull calf), above that of a Holstein bull calf (higher birth BW–lower CED)? Can these data be discovered on a larger farm through data collection and analysis?

DISCLOSURE

The author has no disclosure or conflicts of interest.

REFERENCES

1. Matukumalli LK, Lawley CT, Schnabel RD, et al. Development and characterization of a high density SNP genotyping assay for cattle. PLoS One 2009;4(4):e5350.
2. Guinan FL, Wiggans GR, Norman HD, et al. Changes in genetic trends in US dairy cattle since the implementation of genomic selection. J Dairy Sci 2023;106(2): 1110–29.
3. Berry DP, Wall E, Pryce JE. Genetics and genomics of reproductive performance in dairy and beef cattle. Animal 2014;8(Suppl 1):105–21.
4. Arnold FJ. Fifty Years of D.H.I.A. Work. J Dairy Sci 1956;39(6):792–4.
5. Breeding USCfD. Home page. Available at: https://uscdcb.com.
6. Breeders NAoA. April 2020 Genetic Base Change. 2020. Available at: https://www.naab-css.org/news/april-2020-genetic-base-change. [Accessed 1 April 2024].
7. Norman HD, VanRaden P, Wiggans GR. April 2020: genetic base change. Councin on Dairy Cattle Breeding; 2020. Available at: https://uscdcb.com/wp-content/uploads/2020/02/Norman-et-al-Genetic-Base-Change-April-2020-FINAL_new.pdf. [Accessed 1 April 2024].
8. Norman HD, Wright JR, Hubbard SM, et al. Reproductive status of Holstein and Jersey cows in the United States. J Dairy Sci 2009;92(7):3517–28.
9. Ablondi M, Sabbioni A, Stocco G, et al. Genetic Diversity in the Italian Holstein Dairy Cattle Based on Pedigree and SNP Data Prior and After Genomic Selection. Front Vet Sci 2022;8.
10. Sattler CG. Progeny Testing and Genomics: Where are we and where are we going? Indianapolis, IN: Dairy Cattle Reproduction Conference; 2013.
11. Davenport KM, Spencer JA, Peak JJ, et al. Genomic testing of female Holsteins: a resource for selection and improvement. Transl Anim Sci 2018;2(Suppl 1):S149–54.
12. Wiggans GR, Cole JB, Hubbard SM, et al. Genomic Selection in Dairy Cattle: The USDA Experience. Annu Rev Anim Biosci 2017;5:309–27.
13. CoDC Breeding. CDCB dairy database stats. 2024. Available at: https://uscdcb.com/database-stats. [Accessed 7 March 2024].
14. Holstein Association USA I. Understanding genomic predictions. 2024. Available at: https://www.holsteinusa.com/pdf/print_material/genomics.pdf. [Accessed 7 March 2024].
15. Schulz L. Beef cow herd to shrink for years to come. AgDM Newsletter 2023; 2023:2.
16. United States Department of Agriculture AaPHIS, Veterinary Services, National Animal Health Monitoring System. Beef 2017 beef cow-calf managment practices in the United States 2017 Report 1; 2020.
17. United States Department of Agriculture NASSN. Milk production. 2023. Available at: https://downloads.usda.library.cornell.edu/usda-esmis/files/h989r321c/sb398t09v/w0893v44q/mkpr0923.pdf. [Accessed 1 April 2024].
18. Marrella MA, White RR, Dias NW, et al. Comparison of reproductive performance of AI- and natural service-sired beef females under commercial management. Transl Anim Sci 2021;5(3):txab114.
19. Culbertson R. Beef on Dairy. eBEEF. 2023. Available at: https://ebeef.ucdavis.edu/sites/g/files/dgvnsk7331/files/inline-files/Factsheet2_2023.pdf.
20. (NAAB) NAoAB. Annual reports of semen sales and custom freezing. 2021. Available at: https://www.naab-css.org/semensales.

21. Association AA. EPD and $Value definitions. 2024. Available at: https://www. angus.org/Nce/Definitions. [Accessed 14 March 2024].
22. Touchberry RW, Bereskin B. Crossbreeding Dairy Cattle. I. Some Effects of Crossbreeding on the Birth Weight and Gestation Period of Dairy Cattle1. J Dairy Sci 1966;49(3):287–300.
23. Selk GE, Buchanan DS. Gestation length and birth weight differences of calves born to 9, $^{1}/_{4}$ and ½ blood Brahman fall and spring-calving cows bred to Salers and Limousin sires. 1990. Animal Science Research Reports 1990. Available at: https://extension.okstate.edu/programs/beef-extension/research-reports/site-files/documents/1990/90_3.pdf. [Accessed 14 March 2024].
24. Singh K, Molenaar AJ, Swanson KM, et al. Epigenetics: a possible role in acute and transgenerational regulation of dairy cow milk production. Animal 2012;6(3): 375–81.
25. van Esch BCAM, Porbahaie M, Abbring S, et al. The Impact of Milk and Its Components on Epigenetic Programming of Immune Function in Early Life and Beyond: Implications for Allergy and Asthma. Front Immunol 2020;11:2141.

Role of Veterinary Practitioners in the Genomic Era in Dairy: Economic Impact

Kim Egan, DVM, MBA

KEYWORDS

- Dairy • Genetics • Genomics • Phenotypes • Sustainability

KEY POINTS

- Genetic progress aids in improving dairy and beef herd profitability.
- Veterinarians can assist in gauging the potential impact on overall profitability from implementation of genetic strategies.
- Veterinarians can assess management/environmental impact on epigenetics consultatively and provide solutions to increase herd performance.

As the modern dairy industry focuses on sustainability, the financial margins to continue operating are a primary concern. Large animal veterinarians are acutely aware of consolidation occurring across agriculture driven by a need for efficiency. As veterinarians, it is in our best interest to encourage practices and protocols that add profitability for a herd owner. Our businesses rely on farms and ranches that are financially sustainable. The use of genetic data is a tool to improve profitability—through improved health, fertility, and production efficiency.

As shown in **Fig. 1**,[1] milk production per cow has been steadily increasing in US dairy. An astute veterinarian can analyze genetic progress for production, while also communicating how reducing somatic cell counts or post-fresh health events can help cows to reach their genetic potential for production. In this way, herd veterinarians can use both genetic knowledge and knowledge of a herd's environment and management to maximize phenotypic performance.

Veterinarians who routinely conduct herd health visits can identify opportunities to improve genetic expression through recommendations that improve management. Veterinarians can also coach producers about where genetic focus can be most impactful to reach herd health goals. One example here would be a herd that has inadequate heat abatement for dry cows. There have been numerous presentations based on the work done by Jimena LaPorta and colleagues[2] to show that not only will the daughters of heat-stressed dry cows have poorer immunoglobulin G absorption, lower

Genex Cooperative, 117 East Green Bay Street, Shawano, WI 54166, USA
E-mail address: kegan@genex.coop

Vet Clin Food Anim 40 (2024) 415–421
https://doi.org/10.1016/j.cvfa.2024.05.006
0749-0720/24/© 2024 Elsevier Inc. All rights reserved, including that for text and data mining, AI training, and similar technologies.

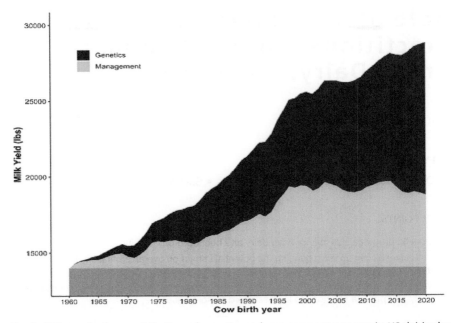

Fig. 1. Milk production contribution of genetics and management per cow in US dairies by birth year.

growth rates, poorer heifer fertility, and reduced production (compared to calves born to cooled cows), but the granddaughters will be similarly affected. The herd veterinarian ideally can consult effectively about epigenetic effects and guide producers to resolve the root causes of the phenotypic expression that are dampening the genetic potential of animals in a herd.

Similarly, maximizing the fertility in a dairy herd will maximize the percentage of cows near peak milk production. Consultation regarding synchronization protocols, breeding equipment, and personnel conducting insemination should all be within the skill set of modern practitioners. **Table 1** shows the difference in conception rates of multiparous cows during their first synchronized breeding. This comparison is within one herd, maintaining consistent environmental, nutritional, and management conditions, and varies by levels of genomic daughter pregnancy rate, a key fertility trait.

High fertility levels, and consequently the percentage of the herd near peak milk, have definite financial advantages. Albert De Vries, of the University of Florida, has analyzed reproductive scenarios demonstrating the impact of fertility on dairy farm economics. He presented data[3] showing that generally there is increased profitability per cow moving to higher pregnancy rates and that beyond 30% to 35% pregnancy rate, there is not considerable additional financial return. Achieving high fertility allows herds to use sexed semen or advanced reproductive techniques with greater success.

Table 1		
Difference in conception rates of multiparous cows by genomic daughter pregnancy rate level		
	GDPR	
	Under 0.2	Over 0.1
First service conception to Double Ovsynch program	47%	55%

(K. Egan.)

Understanding the goals and future vision of dairy and beef producers will align recommendations for successful outcomes. Herd owners who wish to use advanced reproductive techniques, or add certainty to mating strategies, for the improvement of future generations, may consider genomic testing to leverage the accuracy of data in reproductive decision-making.

Genomics gives an indication of the potential outcome of mating—genomic data use the power of gathered data to predict where "daughter proven" would need as many as 15 to 100 offspring for equivalent reliability. Genomics brings the genetic power of the female in line with that which we have historically only given to the sire. Veterinarians can be actively involved in sampling strategies, submissions, and action plans based on results.

GUIDELINES

In the United States, the Department of Agriculture's Council on Dairy Cattle Breeding (CDCB) compiles data from genomic testing and collaborates with official herd testing record centers to produce genetic evaluations. All results are updated in April, August, and December each year. The CDCB uses economic data and trait weights to form the Net Merit $ (NM$) index, along with the Fluid, Cheese, and Grazing Merit $ indexes, each tailored to achieve specific goals of dairy production such as optimizing fluid milk production, cheese yield, or grazing efficiency, respectively.

These metrics are important contributors to composite tools such as the NM$, the Dairy Wellness Profit $, total performance index, and other composite tools that are used by dairy producers to assess the potential monetary value which a heifer might bring to the herd or real monetary value that a cow does give to the herd compared to that female's or male's peers. The formulas are adjusted to reflect real-world cost of production, product value, and genetic "current-ness" of the population of peers. In this way, the formulas remain relevant for comparison. These unseen traits comprise about 47% of the Lifetime Net Merit formula in US dairy cows. If one includes an accurate measure of milk solids yield on a non-lactating heifer, the "unseen" portion of genomic testing on NM$ and other similar formula increases dramatically.

For beef breeds, each breed association publishes data regularly from weekly to monthly.

Base changes occur once every 5 years for dairy breeds, resetting values to compare to the population of a given birth year. For example, currently we are in 2023 comparing to the population born in 2015.

Independent organizations and companies also create customized indexes to adjust to market changes more rapidly than the 5 year window and to adjust weightings for differing markets or include proprietary traits. Some examples include Holstein Association's Total Performance Index, Zoetis' Dairy Wellness Profit $, and GENEX's Ideal Commercial Cow index.

APPLICATION
Genomic Results

As you have read in previous studies, the accuracy of genomic predictions has allowed the identification of high genetic value animals at a very early age. This has shortened the generational interval and accelerated genetic progress. Genomic testing would be worthless without a plan for how the herd will use the results. One example would be using beef semen on the lowest genomic value quartile of the herd, allowing the resulting replacements to have overall higher genetic value. Another strategy involves limiting service with sexed semen to animals with low genomic fertility trait values. A very basic use is to verify sire identification and monitor accuracy in the breeding and maternity data entry.

As genes do not sort equally from gametes, genomic testing can identify outliers that may result from a mating. Herds using advanced reproductive techniques, such as oocyte pick-up, in vitro fertilization, and embryo transfer, can utilize genomic results to identify outliers to propagate or make culling decisions. At the very least, records that include genomic values for the females in a herd may improve the sales value of those females.

After submitting samples to a genomic evaluation laboratory, practitioners can receive results in a spreadsheet format, and/or results can be loaded directly into herd management software or shared via the laboratories Internet platform.

Replacement Strategies

Raising replacement heifers requires an expensive outlay of resources and cash. The use of gender-selected semen, genomic evaluation, and better overall management resulting in lower cull rates has allowed producers to target the females from which they do not wish to have replacement females. An example of these points was a conversation Pat Comyn, DVM had with Gordie Jones, DVM in 2020. The Wisconsin dairy operation they discussed, which Dr Jones was a partner in and managed, had an involuntary cull rate of about 13% to 15% and then had the opportunity to voluntarily cull 15% to 17%. This gives a tremendous opportunity to cut back on a large expenditure—the raising of heifers. The beef x dairy cross calves also brought a greater financial return to the farm than pure dairy bulls.

An example of the difference that can be made in farm income is shown **Table 2**. The changes in breeding strategy and reduction of dairy bull calves being born have improved the 1,200 head dairy farm's income by nearly $100,000 per year versus what it was 5 years ago, based on a modest price per hundredweight of the beef-dairy cross calves.

Impact of Health on Profitability

A practitioner can gain insights into the impact of genetics by assessing differences within herds based on genetics to gauge the impact of genetics given the same management, environment, and nutrition. It is common to see a reduction in transition health events, improvement in reproductive performance, and increased production with higher genetic values. If such differences are imperceptible or nonexistent, this may warrant investigation of management protocols.

Table 2
Income comparison of a dairy farm

Backup Date	August 2023	March 2022	October 2019	October 2018
Sale price of beef cross calf	$150	$130	$130	$150
Sale price of Holstein bull calf	$50	$50	$50	$50
Difference in sold calf price	$100	$80	$80	$100
Number of beef sired calves born alive in last year	997	558	468	170
Number of HO bull calves born alive in last year	58	308	354	708
Sold beef calf sales dollars gained vs dairy bull	$152,450	$87,940	$78,540	$60,900

(K. Egan.)

An example of such an assessment in a group of older cows in one herd is shown in **Table 3**. Comparing cows within one herd helps eliminate the confounding factors of weather-related stress, nutritional differences, or differences in milking procedures or bedding comfort. In this group of second lactation or greater cows, the lowest genetic value quartile of cows has the highest average number of metritis, milk fever, and abortion events. Conversely, the highest genetic value quartile of cows has the lowest average somatic cell count and the fewest days open on average. The cost of days open beyond 90 days in milk has been discussed in several publications, adding to feed cost as the largest expense of operating a dairy farm. As Dr Egan has observed in many herds, the highest genetic value quartile also has the best production in the herd.

FUTURE DIRECTIONS

The largest concern echoed by employers across all industries, especially in animal agriculture, is the availability of labor. Labor is also one of the largest expenses on many dairy farms and beef ranches. To address this, more robotics are being used in dairy herds. In the parlor, or box, we need cows that will function well in the robotic systems that are increasingly being implemented. As mentioned earlier, currently available (in the United States) traits to consider would be moderate body size and correct teat placement and length. In the future, combining milking speed (or box time) with production data will allow robotic herds to build strategies to breed for efficiency.

Nutritional Needs of Global Population

One message that has been repeated in many circles is that the global population is growing and will need more animal protein to thrive. Others have wondered whether we have enough food, but that is just not distributed geographically to meet all needs. In either case, providing high-quality protein to consumers is the main goal of animal agriculture. We must pay attention not only to Predicted Transitting Ability Protein, but to future research on types of protein and sugars in our end products to match and maximize human digestibility function. Another facet to consider for a sustainable future is the water weight in milk being hauled, maximizing components reduces the trucking emissions needed to get dairy products to processing plants. Along with maximizing production, we are on a fixed land base. So, feed efficiency needs to remain a focus. Feed costs can make up over half of the total costs on a dairy farm.[4] Improving the efficiency of dairy cows reduces the amount of natural resources and energy needed to produce and process the feed required for the herd. Also, several studies have shown cows that are more feed efficient also produce lower methane emissions.[5,6]

Table 3							
Assessment of different quartiles of cows from the same herd on different parameters							
Genomic Quartile	Head Count	Average Genomic NM$	Avg. Number of Metritis Events	Avg. Number of Milk Fever Events	Avg. Somatic Cell Count Last Test Day	Avg. Days Open	Avg. Energy-Corrected 305 d Production
1	454	638	1.2	0	106	98	36,357
2	451	512	1.2	0	125	110	35,161
3	454	404	1.1	0	182	116	33,758
4	445	230	1.4	1	215	118	32,054

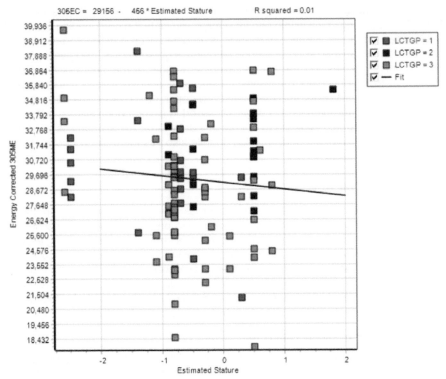

Fig. 2. Average energy-corrected milk production by parent average genetic stature in a single herd. (K. Egan.)

Genetic selection for feed efficiency supports industry goals to reduce the environmental footprint of dairy production.

Income over feed cost (IOFC) is one of the efficiency benchmarks routinely analyzed by lenders and dairy management teams. Obviously, our cows need a good quality, readily available ration to maintain health and productivity. So, in addition to analyzing the ration's components, what other tools can help improve IOFC in long term?

Let us consider feed costs. A readily available good-quality ration is essential. Many producers have looked at the benefits of small-breed cows for their feed efficiency, especially with limits on land availability. Selection for more moderate body size, along with weightings for marginal feed costs and body condition score, can be beneficial in production efficiency. The Nutrient Requirements of Dairy Cattle 2001 formula for estimating dry matter intakes takes body weight into account, larger cows require more dry matter, and increased production also raises dry matter intakes. Jim Linn from the Department of Animal Science at the University of MN simplified these effects by stating that a difference of 100 kg of body weight changes dry matter intake by 1.5 kg/d (3.3 lb/d).[7] How much economic difference does this make? Let us use $0.07 cost per pound of dry matter. A 1,000 cow herd of 1,500 lb Holsteins consumes an average of 52 lb/head/d on a dry matter basis. This would cost $3,640/d. If the same herd had an average body weight of 1,390 lb, the requirement for intakes would decrease to 50.35 lb Dry Matter/head/day, costing $3,524/d. That small difference in body weight would save $42,340 per year on this 1,000 cow example herd. Another, increasingly important, benefit of feed efficiency is the ability to feed more cows with the same land base.

Can cows with lower genetic stature produce as well? Simply, yes. **Fig. 2** depicts average energy-corrected milk production from 134 cows from a single herd with comparable genetic production potential, similar stage of production, housed similarly, subjected to the same milking routine, and fed the same ration. All cows had estimated sire genetic PTA milk between 900 and 1100 and were between 100 and 200 days in milk.

SUMMARY

Genetics plays a crucial role, constituting half of the determinants of herd performance. It serves not only as a tool to address current concerns but also as an opportunity to meet future needs. Veterinarians occupy a unique position to lead in utilizing genetics and genomics to enhance herd profitability and sustainability.

DISCLOSURE

Dr K. Egan is employed by a cooperative primarily involved in genetic sales.

REFERENCES

1. Council on Dairy Cattle Breeding, Impact on US Dairy, Available at: https://uscdcb. com/impact/, 2024. Accessed March 19, 2024.
2. LaPorta J, Ferreira FC, Ouellet V, et al. Late-gestation heat stress impairs daughter and granddaughter lifetime performance. J Dairy Sci 2020;103:7555–68.
3. DeVries A. What is the optimal pregnancy rate? Is being too efficient a benefit or Hindrance? Dairy Cattle Reproduction Council annual meeting 2016.
4. United States Department of Agriculture – Economic Research Service, Milk cost of production estimates, Available at: http://www.ers.usda.gov/data-products/milk-cost-of-production-estimates, 2018. Accessed March 19, 2024.
5. de Haas Y, Windig JJ, Calus MPL, et al. Genetic parameters for predicted methane production and potential for reducing enteric emissions through genomic selection. J Dairy Sci 2011;94:6122–34.
6. Waghorn GC, Hegarty RS. Lowering ruminant methane emissions through improved feed conversion efficiency. Anim Feed Sci Technol 2011;166:291–301.
7. Linn J. Energy in the 2001 Dairy NRC: Understanding the System. Minnesota Dairy Health Conference proceedings 2003.

European Dairy Cattle Evaluations and International Use of Genomic Data

Marco Winters, MSc[a],*, Mike Coffey, PhD[b], Raphael Mrode, PhD[b]

KEYWORDS

- INTERBULL • Genotypes • Phenotypes • Evaluations • Breeding

KEY POINTS

- Dairy cattle evaluations in Europe are dispersed and mainly operate at national, individual country level.
- International collaboration and sharing of phenotypes and genotypes increase the accuracy and usefulness of genetic evaluations.
- Breeding requirements are shifting toward lowering cost and improving environmental sustainability and, as a result, require new phenotypes to be recorded which are often expensive.
- Dairy cattle breeding companies increasingly are multinationals, and fierce competition is encouraging proprietary phenotype collection and in-house evaluations, putting constraints on the sharing of data.
- New ways of collaborating to maintain evaluation accuracies and global comparisons need to be explored, to continue to provide the success that dairy cattle breeding has enjoyed over many decades.

INTRODUCTION

The continent of Europe consists of 44 countries, operating dairy cattle breeding largely as independent countries, and has a diverse range of dairy cattle breeds, with the Holstein being the predominant breed. The genetic evaluations of European dairy cattle are similarly numeric and dispersed. Each individual country typically operates its own national evaluation center, which is responsible for collating the national phenotypes, pedigrees, and genotypes to conduct the animal evaluations and produce estimated breeding values (EBVs).

---

[a] AHDB - Agriculture and Horticulture Development Board, Coventry, UK; [b] Livestock Informatics, Animal Breeding and Genomics Team, SRUC – Scotland's Rural College, Edinburgh, UK
* Corresponding author. AHDB, Middlemarch Business Park, Siskin Parkway East, Coventry CV3 4PE, UK.
E-mail address: Marco.winters@ahdb.org.uk

Vet Clin Food Anim 40 (2024) 423–434
https://doi.org/10.1016/j.cvfa.2024.05.007
0749-0720/24/© 2024 Elsevier Inc. All rights reserved, including those for text and data mining, AI training, and similar technologies.

Despite the national focus, for some populations, there are cross-border evaluations. Examples of these are the Fleckvieh evaluations of Austria and German populations that are evaluated as one. Similarly, the Scandinavian countries Denmark, Sweden, and Finland have pooled their data and evaluations. But for the majority of breeds and countries, each country still carries out its own.

In order to compare and convert these evaluations from the various centers across Europe, and elsewhere, onto a comparable scale, the International Bull Evaluation Service (INTERBULL) was established in 1983 as a Permanent Sub-Committee of The International Committee for Animal Recording.

INTERBULL uses a method referred to as multitrait across country evaluation (MACE) to combine EBVs from several countries into a single international evaluation. MACE is based on the multitrait best linear unbiased prediction (BLUP) method described by Schaeffer[1] and regards EBVs for the same trait from different countries as different traits. This allows MACE to account for differences among countries in the heritability of the trait and the way the traits are measured, or differences in scale. MACE estimates the genetic correlations among the countries based on the genetic links among the participating countries, and these correlations are incorporated in calculating the genetic merit of bulls on the international scale. These genetic correlations also account for any genotype-by-environment interaction, for example, for the same milk production trait in countries with very different management systems. The international evaluations are produced and expressed for each sire on the local scale of the different countries and are usually of higher accuracy compared to national evaluations as information from daughters in all countries are utilized. Currently, MACE is based on data from 35 countries and is carried out 3 times per year (https://interbull.org/ib/users_map).

Thus, INTERBULL fulfills an important role in the validation and comparison of international breeding values for its member organizations. A major output of this process is the ability to compare bulls across countries even when no daughters are milking in a particular country. This provides an international benchmark for participating countries and the ability for farmers to make informed choices on daughter-proven artificial insemination (AI) bulls irrespective of the country of origin of the bull. This enables the local farmers to tap into a global resource of unbiased ranked bulls, enabling stronger selection intensity and a higher accuracy of EBVs to select from.

The origins of INTERBULL lie in an era where compute resources were very expensive, and so it was infeasible for countries to share raw phenotypes for INTERBULL to calculate international evaluations. Instead, bull proofs were deregressed and effectively became the phenotype used in the international evaluations (in essence the "average" daughter of each bull corrected for all locally known effects). This was computationally more feasible in the timeframe required and at a cost that most countries find acceptable.

An important point to note is that the service users of INTERBULL, and as such the evaluation units conducting the analysis, operate as impartial and independent organizations whose sole aim is to provide accurate and unbiased ranking of dairy cattle. Although some contributions are made by commercial breeding companies toward the activities of the national evaluation units, on the whole, the activities are financed from contributions of national governments and/or farmers.

TRANSITION FROM PHENOTYPIC TO GENOMIC EVALUATIONS

Genetic evaluations in the dairy industry have for decades been heavily reliant on the analysis of very large quantities of phenotypic performance records recorded by farmers for the purposes of farm management. The strong co-operative mentality among the various stakeholders has provided a valuable collective resource for farmers and breeding organizations alike. These many millions of performance records, alongside pedigree records, have enabled highly reliable genetic assessments of individuals to be made, in particular for sires with many progeny. The exchange of pedigree data among countries has enabled each national evaluation to run with the most accurate pedigree leading to higher accuracy EBVs.

Genomic evaluation, where genetic assessments are made based on the animals' single nucleotide polymorphism (SNP) profile, derived from their DNA, and phenotypic information, rather than phenotype and pedigree alone have dramatically changed the dairy breeding industries since 2009.[2] The availability of low-cost genotyping prompted a quick uptake by many countries and breeding companies to genotype their most prolific breeding bulls, followed by those daughter-proven sires that still had DNA available (mostly in the form of frozen semen). Daughter-proven sires were the first group of animals to be genotyped initially, as genomic evaluations rely firstly on establishing a reference population of individuals that have both genotypes and performance data available. And the greatest value is derived from those individuals who have a high-accuracy phenotype. To this end, sires that have 1000s of progeny end up being the most informative. However, early excitement soon turned into a reality check that the systems require many 1000s of high accuracy genotyped individuals to gain higher genomic accuracy predictions.[3] Research also quickly revealed that to maximize the value of the genomic insight, the reference population needed to be related as close as possible to the candidate animals that were being genotyped today. In practical terms, this means that the youngest generation of proven bulls for the breed of interest need to be in the reference, and more recently, performance-recorded female individuals have additionally fulfilled this need.

Changes to the historic contributors of data started to happen when genomics became widely adopted. Unlike the phenotypic resource data, which have largely been paid for by farmers, primarily for farm management purposes, the genotypic data were, to a large extent, funded by commercial breeding companies looking to accelerate the genetic gains their programs could deliver with this new genomic knowledge. This changed the dynamics of co-operation between countries and made many countries very protective of their genotype resources. And since genomic prediction accuracy relies on the combination of both genotype and phenotype, the protection of valuable phenotypes has also become greater.

INTERNATIONAL USE OF GENOMIC DATA

Because most countries have finite resources to build large enough reference populations by themselves (both phenotypes and genotypes, but also financial), genomic evaluations ultimately encouraged groups of countries to collaborate. The sharing arrangements that were formed initially were largely restricted to equal-sized, or likeminded, breeding operators and countries leading to the formation of 2 large international consortia, established to exchange Holstein genotype information. Six European countries formed the EuroGenomics cooperative in 2009 to share Holstein bull genotypes (https://www.eurogenomics.com/). EuroGenomics has expanded since the launch to 10 member countries today. At the same time, the North American consortium between Canada and the United States materialized, and fairly quickly extended to incorporate the United Kingdom and Italy.

Unlike the Holstein breed, the international Brown Swiss herdbooks opted to join forces globally and pool all their male genotypes through the InterGenomics portal managed by INTERBULL.[4] The sharing of genotypes enabled each country to enhance their local predictions, but using genotypes on the male individuals, and the MACE or locally calculated EBVs.

A similar service has since expanded to the Holstein breed for countries that are not part of the 2 large consortia mentioned previously, and who have a common goal of increasing their genomic prediction accuracies.[5] However, this service is purely based on providing genomic-enhanced breeding values and does not share genotypes with all participants.

The genomic evaluation method of most countries is still based on a 2 step approach. This implies that in the first step, each country implements their national genetic evaluations based on phenotypes and pedigrees using various standard BLUP models. The bull proofs (or EBVs) from the national genetic evaluation are then sent to INTERBULL to be used in MACE as described earlier. In the second step, the foreign MACE bull proofs received back from INTERBULL by each country, as well as the national EBVs for local bulls are deregressed and used as input variables for the genomic evaluation systems. In some countries, cows are also included in the reference of the genomic systems, and in this case, the yield deviation of cows (phenotypes corrected for known fixed effects) are used as input variables. The input variables (phenotypes and pedigree) are then used together with the genotypes of animals in the reference to compute SNP effects and direct genomic values (DGVs) for animals. Given that national genomic evaluations are based on a subset of animals that have phenotypes, it ignores additional information from the pedigree and phenotypes of related nongenotyped animals. To overcome this, this additional information is combined with the DGVs using a selection index approach to produce the genomic breeding values (GEBVs) for animals, which are the figures published and used by the industry to assess the genetic merit of selection candidates.[6]

As indicated, this 2 step approach implies that genotyped animals are a subset of the entire population, and these could potentially be preferentially selected. In addition, the reference population over time will only include young bulls that are of high performance and therefore have been highly preselected based on their genomic evaluations, derived from their SNP profile. This, therefore, over time introduces a selection bias in the genomic evaluation based on the 2 step approach.

This limitation with the 2 step approach led to the development of the 1 step approach (or single step) that involves the computation of GEBVs through the combined use of nongenotyped and genotyped animals together in a single evaluation model.[7] This involves using phenotypes and pedigree information for all animals and genotypes for all genotyped animals in an evaluation model, which incorporates the genetic relations of all animals through the use of a so-called H matrix. This enables the flow of information from genotyped animals to nongenotyped animals and vice versa. The inclusion of all genotyped animals in the evaluation overcomes some of the selection bias associated with the 2 step approach and results in higher accuracies overall.

The role of INTERBULL remains important even in these single-step models, as deregressed MACE EBVs are used as input phenotypes for foreign bulls. This group of bulls still constitutes a major part of the input to genomic models of most countries.

At INTERBULL level the implementation of single-step approach faces the same challenges as the 2 step approach due to the sensitivity of exchanging genotypes.

It is widely accepted that a 1 step process of genomic evaluation makes better use of all information and leads to higher accuracy evaluations. Better still would be an international sharing of all data to perform a global genomic evaluation. Such a global single-step dairy evaluation would entail collecting hundreds of millions of individual animal records from all over the world, with associated genotypes to allow the computation to take place in one central location. Even with modern computing power, this would still result in unacceptable slow running times. The size and scope of the problem have led to alternative strategies being suggested such as the exchange of SNP key solutions from individual countries for the creation of a single international SNP key (SNP-MACE).[8] This would not require all phenotype and genotype data to be shared. Although this would pave the way for higher reliability genomic estimates for all countries involved, the logistical issues and problems of exchanging very commercially important data from a range of data suppliers means this option is still being researched and discussed.

For now, bilateral sharing of genotypes from marketed bulls has widely been established among countries. This process enables the local evaluation units to process the information of the genotype and provide genomic predictions on the local base and scale using the local SNP solutions. Alongside elite male individuals, the incorporation of their dam genotypes in single-step genomics might further drive the exchange of genotypes globally.

#PHENOTYPEISKING

With the introduction of genomic evaluations, the reliance on, and use of phenotypes has changed but has certainly not diminished.[9] Initial suggestions[10] that recording costs would decline by 90% have not materialized because phenotypes still need to be collected on animals in the reference by somebody. The belief that genomic information would eliminate the need to record performance data was quickly set straight. More than ever, the breeding industry relies on phenotypes not only to perform the initial calibration and validation but also to perform continued recalibration of the SNP-key to maintain its predictive capability. However, the requirement of mass recording by farmers for genetic selection has reduced somewhat, and many breeding companies have begun funding the collection of new phenotypes important to their own breeding programs instead. Examples are feed intake, methane emissions, and specific disease traits. These commercial phenotypes are mostly not shared with national evaluation units but are used to estimate proprietary GEBVs by breeding companies instead.

The interest in recording new trait phenotypes by the breeding companies is typically motivated by the desire to both increase market share and to maintain unique selling points of their bulls, in an era where many of the top International Holsteins originate from similar bloodlines. This has led to nucleus herds recording traits like feed intake and methane emissions on specific bulls' daughters. Sometimes these nucleus herds will be those owned by the breeding companies and other times herds contracted by them to produce phenotypes. These are sometimes referred to as "phenotype farms" as they are farming phenotypes as an additional source of revenue thereby allowing the breeding companies to generate data on commercial farms but, at the same time, ensuring competitors do not get access to the data. These proprietary GEBVs produced in-house by the breeding companies are rapidly altering the makeup of data sets used in national evaluations that have traditionally been based on data on all animals freely available. It is unknown which evaluations include a subset of new data on specific animals "owned" by the breeding companies.

GENE FLOW

The rapid and wide-spread adoption of genomic evaluation has been remarkable. In only a short time since its introduction in 2009, the developed world has now made genomic predictions commonplace. In many countries, the use of genomic young sires, in preference to older daughter-proven sires, dominates breeding decisions, and genomic testing of female individuals is also practiced widely.[11]

This uptake has accelerated genetic gains in these populations, and continues to not only benefit the users of these tools but also assists the global desire to improve efficiency and reduce greenhouse gases.[12]

However, these more rapid genetic gains also increase inbreeding as the global breeding population becomes more related, due to widespread global use of top-ranking sires.[13] Note this increase in inbreeding is not an automatic outcome of genomic selection, merely an accelerated outcome based on the competition between breeding companies to market the highest merit bulls, largely sourced from similar pedigree ancestors. The international flow of, and insight into, genomic information for selection candidates and an across breeding company collaboration, on selecting bulls for marketing could alleviate that problem but is unlikely to occur due to the free market operating in most countries and the fiercely competitive nature of the breeding companies.

FUTURE DIRECTIONS

Changes to the dairy cattle breeding sector since the introduction of genomics continue to evolve. The major breeding companies are operating globally, rather than nationally, and many of these now operate their own female nucleus herds. The importance of owning not only the leading sires but also the leading female individuals regained importance with the introduction of genomics. The fact that the accuracy of the genomic test is the same in both male and female individuals enables early breeding decisions to be made in both sexes. Owning elite female individuals enables breeding companies to control and protect their genetic superiority and is leading to "lines" being developed by breeding companies, similar to that seen in the pig and poultry breeding schemes. In addition, the use of sexed semen and contractual intellectual property (IP) protection of genetic material further reinforces this breeding structure. In addition, the introduction of proprietary genetic evaluations belonging to the individual companies means that provision of independent genetic and genomic evaluations by national evaluation centers, as has been the case for previous decades, is no longer the sole source of information for farmers. With the dairy farmer in mind as the ultimate customer, it has yet to be determined what the optimum mix of these independent versus proprietary evaluations will be.

However, even in an alternate future, the need for (inter)national collaboration among the many stakeholders remains critical for the foreseeable future, especially for traits like methane emissions that are a global, not local, issue. Existing datasets are needed for continuing evaluations and enhancement of models, and new processes could extract more information from the same existing data. For new and novel traits, it can be envisaged that individual breeding companies will develop their own source of data and produce proprietary indices relating only to their own bulls. This means comparisons between bulls across breeding companies for these new trait evaluations will not be able to be made anymore, but the competition among companies is likely to mean that all bulls will, in any case, be better than that which could be produced by poorly resourced national recording programs. The INTERBULL membership may also evolve, with breeding companies supplying their proprietary evaluations to INTERBULL to enable international rankings to be produced. This new dynamic is happening at a time when, increasingly, governments are becoming more interested in the role of farmed livestock not only because of food security and food safety but also because of the impact that livestock farming has on national carbon emissions.

For the last 70 or so years, European agriculture has developed to feed everyone and produce food at low prices in a consistent way. However, it has become clear that this policy has come at the cost of the variety of ecosystems that society is now valuing more highly. Examples are environmental damage, loss of biodiversity, and disposal of farm waste. This change in attitude to the way food is produced is having an impact on farmers through the retailers who are (apparently) acting as the voice of the consumer. Standards of production are being introduced that have no legal basis but result from society establishing a "license to produce," which suggests that not just the cost of food is important. This will change the type of cow that will be bred, the range of phenotypes needed to support that change and the types of farming practices to produce food that meets that license to produce.

A number of examples are obvious.

Feed Efficiency

The historically relatively low price of energy has led to its increased use on farm and resulted in increasingly marginal improvements in profitability. Increasing yields with associated lower fertility and poorer survival led to the introduction in most countries of indices to counter these unwanted correlated responses. Each incremental unit of input resulted in less than one unit of incremental output but the maintenance feed cost of the cow was diluted by this increased output supported by cheap energy inputs. The recent price spike in energy resulting from geopolitical events worldwide has refocused farming on resource use efficiency across all cost items. Given that feed costs represent over 60% of input costs it follows that careful use of expensive inputs will follow.

Antibiotic Use

The routine use of antibiotics at drying off has reduced considerably as farmers realize that the convenience of dosing every cow is a socially expensive risk and does not fit with the emerging trends in license to produce. This makes selection for reduced mastitis a higher priority than it has been in the past.

Lameness

The prevalence of lameness in dairy cows is estimated at 22%.[14] This is undesirable for production and fertility, and most farmers give lameness a high degree of attention on farm. However, society views lameness as unacceptable and the pressure from lobby groups is a zero tolerance to lameness. This again implies a higher proportion of selection pressure in the future. This will require large numbers of high-accuracy lameness phenotypes to support that evaluation and data collected by professional foot trimmers may be increasingly used.

Methane Emissions

This trait has arguably the highest attention at the moment and is currently the most difficult and expensive trait to measure. A lot of research is underway internationally to find alternative and proxy measures of methane emission that can be used both in national genetic evaluations and in carbon audit tools increasingly being deployed to monitor environmental impact of farms.

As the number of traits evaluated increases and the volume of data available increases, the methods for handling, processing, and evaluating will have to change as well. Current systems of genomic evaluation are complex and mature and have been built up over the last 15 years to run routinely and as fast as needed. However, with the impending availability of automation in phenotype collection, a tsunami of data is heading our way. This means increased attention will have to be paid to data handling methods before genetic evaluation. Historically, many centers have simply bought more and more compute power, more random access memory (RAM), and disc space to keep up with demand. It is unlikely that this approach will be economically able to keep pace with future data supply, and so alternative strategies will need to be developed. This will include rewriting existing systems to be more efficient in function by using different processing strategies, using hardware more effectively, for example, graphics processing units (GPUs), and filtering data to include only that which has information content.

MACHINE LEARNING

Like other industries, cattle breeding is starting to explore the potential that machine learning and artificial intelligence are unlocking. For genetic and genomic evaluations, the real breakthroughs are yet to be unlocked, but for phenotype generation, these tools are already starting to be exploited.

Machine learning is particularly good at using information from images. As such, there is a large effort underway in using digital image capture and automated feature extraction to create new phenotypes. An example of this is CattleEye (CattleEye, Belfast), which uses conventional digital cameras to remotely capture lameness information.[15] Goat udder scores have been automatically extracted from images collected at milking on a rotary parlor.[16] There are products that use images to predict liveweight, which offers the opportunity to gather liveweights on millions of cattle and in dairy cattle, the important change in liveweight over lactation. Similarly, prototypes for an automated type classification system are being developed allowing farmers to classify their own cattle using an app on a mobile phone, thereby doing away with the expense of sending trained classifiers around the country with the associated economic and environmental costs (https://www.iclassifier.ca).

There has been a large global effort over the last 10 or so years to further utilize the milk mid-infrared (MIR) spectral data produced by milk analyzers and used to predict fat and protein percentage in milk. These data were previously viewed as a by-product (waste) of the process and deleted after prediction. Research has been ongoing to predict a wider range of phenotypes from the same spectral data with some success (fatty acids and lactoferrin,[17,18] energy balance, nonesterified fatty acids [NEFA], β-hydroxybutyrate [BHB],[19] and methane).[20] Many are attempting to predict feed intake from milk MIR and some are looking for signals associated with pregnancy and bovine tuberculosis (bTB).[21,22] These phenotype predictions rely on having a set of phenotypes and MIR spectral data on reference animals. The process is like genomic prediction in that a core group of well-recorded animals create a prediction equation that can be applied to a far bigger dataset of animals with spectral data but without the phenotype—coining the phrase "freenotypes."

Despite the exciting opportunities and promising new ways of recording, the requirement for a well-phenotyped, expensive reference population for genomic selection remains. These can either be established locally or pooled globally to improve prediction accuracies. But whereas this sharing may have been common practice in the past, it is likely to continue to be more restricted in the new genomics era.

FUTURE BREEDING GOALS ENABLED BY DATA EXCHANGE

Despite a much better, and much earlier, assessment of the bovine genetic makeup through genomics and increasingly more complex systems to generate and analyze phenotypes, the basic principle of sound selection strategies still starts with understanding the requirements of the future dairy industry.

For this, national breeding goals still play a crucial role. Despite breeding companies becoming more globally focused, the local environmental, political, and societal pressures to respond to local signals remain very important and are likely best served by national breeding goals supported by national breeding values that allow all farmers to make informed, unbiased decisions to suit their own markets and circumstances.

There are, however, common threads appearing. Environmental sustainability is arguably the strongest most recent signal that the dairy breeding sector, like society as a whole, is trying to tackle. Many of the genetic indices already contribute not only to improved financial but also to environmental sustainability. For the last 3 decades, there has been a gradual shift away from a focus on production output, toward reduced costs.[23] Improved genetics for health, fertility, and longevity have already benefited the dairy industry. In more recent years, several countries have introduced feed efficiency evaluations to reduce inputs further.[24] Direct indicators and indices directly aimed at environmental sustainability have started to appear since about 2020.[25,26]

With higher uptake of sexed semen (84% in the United Kingdom; https://ahdb.org.uk/news/survey-reveals-a-significant-increase-in-sexed-dairy-semen), we are also seeing an increase in the use of beef sires in the dairy herd. This is leading to the dairy herd becoming more important to the beef supply chain as well.[27]

BEEF FROM DAIRY AND SIZE OF DAIRY COWS

Previous selection policies by both farmers and breeding companies have led to an increase in the size of the average dairy cows. The increased focus on costs and especially resource use efficiency has more recently caused farmers to begin reducing cow size.

In countries where extensive use of sexed semen is made in the dairy herd, a larger proportion of cows are inseminated to beef bulls and as such a greater proportion of national beef output is from dairy cows. If dairy cows reduce in size to become more efficient, then beef output may consequently reduce. However, the overall efficiency of both industries is important at a national level and so may require some government intervention to ensure the equitable spread of risk and reward across the converging dairy and beef industries. At present, the beef value of the calf is exploited by the grower and finisher with little market signal to the dairy farmer to use a good beef bull. Pregnancy and easy calving are the goals for dairy farmers.

Just as the global gene-flow of elite dairy semen has evolved, it is not unlikely that a similar evolution will emerge for beef genetics for use in the dairy herd. This global flow of genetic material for beef is in its infancy but, due to similar arguments as addressed in this study (eg, genotyping, phenotyping costs), will almost certainly grow. An example is Interbeef that undertakes international evaluation of beef bulls. Recently that has included carcass traits so bulls can be compared internationally for their offspring carcass characteristics further enabling dairy and beef producers to optimize across both sectors.[28]

DISCUSSION

Genomic selection has been an outstanding success and has delivered large benefits to dairy farmers in those industrialized dairying nations that have the financial and logistical infrastructure to exploit the technology. Most traits that were of previous economic significance now have GEBVs calculated that deliver the benefits. It has changed the way breeding companies procure bulls to go into AI and has begun to change the way phenotypes are collected, curated, and shared as the new traits begin to be exploited.

Examples of those traits include feed intake or an efficiency-derived measure, methane emissions, calf and cow survival, and disease resistance, all of which are (or soon will be) cost items on the balance sheet. Since genotyping is now routine and relatively cheap, large numbers have been gathered, and increasingly dairy herds are genotyping all young calves. However, those rare and expensive (and valuable) phenotypes are now becoming the focus of attention in many countries because an SNP key can retrospectively predict for animals without phenotypes, including historically phenotyped and now dead animals, allowing the monitoring of genetic trends for the new trait.

Crossbreeding is routine in pig and poultry breeding and is used extensively in beef and lamb production. However, it has not really yet impacted significantly in dairy since progress in the main breeds (especially Holstein) has limited its appeal. Crossbreeding may increase in popularity once across-breed genomic evaluations are widely and routinely available since crossbred cows are generally smaller and may be better suited to emerging economic circumstances focusing on resource use efficiency, especially fossil fuels. The use of genotypes to check for parentage errors and to assign parentage enables crossbreds to have a certified pedigree. Perhaps, in the future, when all animals are genotyped, the industry will move toward "genotype societies" rather than breed societies where particular genotypes are the favored trait rather than any specific color, shape, or heritage.

A number of initiatives have begun on international collaboration in collecting methane phenotypes (https://www.wur.nl/en/research-results/research-institutes/livestock-research/show-wlr/5-million-grant-for-breeding-efforts-to-reduce-methane.htm). This is a logical undertaking meaning that internationally we can globally reduce methane emissions much quicker. However, it is not obvious how it would fit in with individual collaborating breeding companies wishing to establish a unique selling point. Perhaps, global methane emissions are bigger than global breeding companies?

It is conceivable that rising costs and lower societal acceptance of fossil fuel-derived energy will lead to even faster and more radical changes in data sharing, particularly for resource use traits. The last 70 years have seen the globalization of breeding companies with ever more focus on standardized and proprietary products. This has led to arguably the best cows ever bred for milk production under the economic circumstances that have prevailed. One scenario for future breeding is that the process will simply continue at an accelerated pace based on competition among breeding companies, leading to ever improving cows.

An alternative scenario for the future is that "society" will impose demands on dairy production and breeding that do not lend themselves well to the market forces approach and so some government intervention may increase. A variant of that is retailers intervene "on behalf" of consumers to further impose breeding and production standards. These scenarios will be further complicated by the varying legislative approaches taken worldwide to new genetic technologies such as gene editing. How will superior gene-edited genetic material be used "fairly" to improve lives and reduce environmental impact? How will offspring of edited animals find their way into other markets? How will the products of edited animals be traded and controlled? These are scenarios yet to be played out in a world where technology is advancing faster than the legislation required to protect consumers while encouraging innovation.

DISCLOSURE

The authors are all fully funded by their own organisations and received no funding from commercial companies for this work.

REFERENCES

1. Schaeffer LR. Multiple-country comparison of dairy sires. J Dairy Sci 1994;77: 2671–8.
2. INTERBULL, 2009. Proceedings of the Interbull technical workshop; Genomic Information in Genetic evaluations. No.39.
3. Goddard ME, Hayes BJ, Meuwissen THE. Using the genomic relationship matrix to predict accuracy of genomic selection. Journal of animal breeding and genetics = Zeitschrift für Tierzüchtung und Züchtungsbiologie 2011;128:409–21.
4. Jorjani Hossein, Jakobsen Jette, Nilforooshan Mohammad, et al. Genomic Evaluation of BSW Populations InterGenomics: Results and Deliverables. Interbull Bulletin 2011;43.
5. Savoia, S. (2021). Interbull genomic evaluation of small Holstein populations: InterGenomics-Holstein (IG-HOL). INTERBULL BULLETIN NO. 56.
6. VanRaden PM. Efficient methods to compute genomic predictions. J Dairy Sci 2008;91:4414–23.
7. Misztal I, Aguilar I, Legarra A, et al. A unified approach to utilize phenotypic, full pedigree and genomic information for genetic evaluation. Leipzig, Germany: Proceedings of the 9th world congress applied to livestock production; 2010. Communication no. 0050.
8. Goddard, M.E., A. Jighly, H. Benhajali, H. Jorjani and Z. Liu.(2018). SNPMace – A meta-analysis to estimate SNP effects by combining results from multiple countries. INTERBULL BULLETIN NO. 54.
9. Coffey M. Dairy cows: in the age of the genotype, #phenotypeisking. Animal Frontiers 2020;10(2):19–22.
10. Schaeffer LR. Strategy for applying genome-wide selection in dairy cattle. J Anim Breed Genet 2006;123:218–23.
11. Wiggans GR, Cole JB, Hubbard SM, et al. Genomic Selection in Dairy Cattle: The USDA Experience. Annual Review of Animal Biosciences 2017;5(1):309–27.
12. Pryce JE, Mekonnen Haile-Mariam M. Symposium review: Genomic selection for reducing environmental impact and adapting to climate change. J Dairy Sci 2020;103:5366–75.
13. Cole JB. Perspective: Can we actually do anything about inbreeding? J Dairy Sci 2024;107(2):643–8.
14. Thomsen PT, Shearer JK, Houe H. Prevalence of lameness in dairy cows: A literature review. Vet J 2023;295:105975.
15. Anagnostopoulos A, Griffiths BE, Siachos N, et al. Initial validation of an intelligent video surveillance system for automatic detection of dairy cattle lameness. Front Vet Sci 2023;10:1111057.
16. Robson J, Denholm S, Coffey M. Automated Processing and phenotype extraction of Ovine Medical images using a combined generative Adversarial Network and Computer Vision Pipeline. Sensors 2021;21(21):7268.
17. Soyeurt H, Dehareng F, Gengler N, et al. Mid-infrared prediction of bovine milk fatty acids across multiple breeds, production systems, and countries. J Dairy Sci 2011;94(Issue 4):1657–67.

18. Soyeurt H, Grelet C, McParland S, et al. A comparison of 4 different machine learning algorithms to predict lactoferrin content in bovine milk from mid-infrared spectra. J Dairy Sci 2020;103(12):11585–96.
19. Smith SL, Denholm SJ, Coffey MP, et al. Energy profiling of dairy cows from routine milk mid-infrared analysis. J Dairy Sci 2019;102(12):11169–79.
20. Dehareng F, Delfosse C, Froidmont E, et al. Potential use of milk mid-infrared spectra to predict individual methane emission of dairy cows. Animal 2012; 6(23031566):1694–701.
21. Brand W, Wells AT, Smith SL, et al. Predicting pregnancy status from mid-infrared spectroscopy in dairy cow milk using deep learning. J Dairy Sci 2021;104(4): 4980–90.
22. Denholm SJ, Brand W, Mitchell AP, et al. Predicting bovine tuberculosis status of dairy cows from mid-infrared spectral data of milk using deep learning. J Dairy Sci 2020;103(10):9355–67.
23. Miglior F, Fleming A, Malchiodi F, et al. A 100-Year Review: Identification and genetic selection of economically important traits in dairy cattle. J Dairy Sci 2017; 100(12):10251–71.
24. Li B, Mrode R, Id-Lahoucine S, et al. Genomic Evaluation for Feed Advantage–Towards Feed Efficient Cows in UK Dairy Cattle. Interbull Bulletin 2021;56:125–30.
25. Winters M, Coffey M. The EnviroCow index and its impact on the UK dairy industry's carbon footprint. Interbull Bulletin 2023;59:83–8.
26. Richardson CM, Amer PR, Quinton C, et al. Reducing greenhouse gas emissions through genetic selection in the Australian dairy industry. J Dairy Sci 2022;105(5): 4272–88.
27. Newton J, Shaffer M, Cromie A. Beef from Dairy: The role of genetic improvement in creating greater integration between our dairy and beef industries. ICAR proceedings. Toledo 2023.
28. Macedo F. International beef evaluations for Carcass traits. Interbull bulletin 2023; 59:197–201.

The Benefit of a National Genomic Testing Scheme

Donagh P. Berry, PhD, MSc Bioinformatics, BAgrSc[a],*,
Matthew L. Spangler, PhD, MSc, BSc (Anim Sci)[b]

KEYWORDS

- Genotype • Cattle • Sheep • Single nucleotide polymorphism • Parentage
- Genomic evaluation

KEY POINTS

- Individual animal genotypes, especially as part of a national genotyping initiative, provide valuable information to help inform value-creating breeding and management decisions.
- By having all animals in a population genotyped for several thousand DNA markers, the parents of each animal can be automatically detected if all data are stored centrally; any biological sample can also be traced back to an individual.
- The larger the population of genotyped animals with performance information, the greater the accuracy of the resulting predictions of genetic merit; this is especially true for traits less under genetic control (ie, low heritability).
- Accurate prediction of genetic merit enables more precise management decisions such as the grouping of homogenous animals for management purposes, identification of high somatic cell count animals from bulk milk tank genotypes, and the decision to alter animal performance thresholds to trigger mitigation/remedial action based on the (estimated) genetic susceptibility of the individual.

INTRODUCTION

The use of genomic information in ruminant populations is not new. DNA has been used in ruminant populations to verify parentage since the 1990s; such assessments were generally confined to only high-value animals like those used in artificial insemination or registered in breed societies. The approach used when originally deployed was based on microsatellite technology which, although accurate, could not always be fully automated resulting in it being cumbersome and costly due, in part, to a slow throughput rate. Implementing a national genotyping strategy using microsatellites would have required considerable resources and, other than their use to verify parentage, the additional benefits nationally would have been relatively small.

[a] Animal & Grassland Research and Innovation Centre, Teagasc, Moorepark, Fermoy, Cork, P61 C996, Ireland; [b] Department of Animal Science, University of Nebraska-Lincoln, Lincoln, NE, USA
* Corresponding author.
E-mail address: donagh.berry@teagasc.ie

Vet Clin Food Anim 40 (2024) 435–445
https://doi.org/10.1016/j.cvfa.2024.05.008

Marker-assisted selection using a few genetic markers was commercialized in cattle in the early 2000s. Slight improvements in the accuracy of predicting the genetic merit of individuals were reported.[1] It soon became apparent, however, that the predictions of performance for quantitative traits based on a limited number of genetic markers did not always perform well across family lines[2]; single marker tests for mono-genetically or oligogenetically inherited traits (eg, congenital defects, double muscling, fecundity, lethal mutations) still had utility. Nonetheless, the applicability, and therefore usefulness, of such low-density genetic marker tests as part of a whole population genotyping strategy was limited.

In order, therefore, for a national genotyping scheme to be justified, several criteria should be fulfilled.

- The acquisition of a biological sample should not be overly cumbersome.
- There should be a return-on-investment in the initiative which, in itself would be conditional on
  - A relatively low cost of the entire genotyping service from sample to result.
  - The genotype data generated should ideally solve multiple problem statements and the information should be provided in a readily useable form.
- The necessary infrastructure should be in place to be able to handle the samples and resulting genomic data and convert it into information for the end user.
- The knowledge should exist within the sector to be able to properly interpret and advise on the generated information.
- The information provided to the client should be acted upon.

Access to a low-cost genotyping platform that could generate sufficient, accurate (ie, repeatable), and informative genotypes became a reality with the commercial availability of dense genotype panels. The genotype density panel most commonly used in most ruminant populations globally consists of circa 50,000 tiny DNA variants (called single nucleotide polymorphisms or SNPs). These platforms are referred to as SNP-chips and are discussed in detail elsewhere[3]; there is a movement beginning to transition from the current SNP-chips to sequencing approaches with only a part of the genome being sequenced (ie, low-pass sequence). Irrespective of technology, however, the output is generally the same—genotypes on tens if not hundreds of thousands of locations in the genome.

This article focuses on many of the applications of genotype data in ruminant production systems all of which are discussed in detail elsewhere[4]; the emphasis in this article is the applications that benefit most from a national genotyping program.

Parentage

The estimated genetic merit of an individual at birth is simply the average of the respective genetic merit estimates of the parents; the accuracy (reliability) of that genetic evaluation is the sum of half (quarter) the reliability of the sire and dam. Knowing parentage (and by extension, relationships) is also important to help determine the expected co-ancestry between candidate mates which equates to the expected inbreeding of the potential offspring. Where the breed composition of the candidate parents is known, then the expected heterosis of the offspring can also be established. With traditional genetic evaluations, missing parentage and to a greater extent incorrect parentage records have repercussions for genetic gain.[5] The higher the rate of parentage errors, the greater the impact on genetic gain.[5] Where mob mating exists (eg, beef rangelands or sheep), it is often not feasible to record mating events for inferring parentage. The dilemma is especially exacerbated in polyovulatory species where superfecundation may occur. Using a population of 539 pairs of genotyped twins lambs born to mob mating with genotyped rams, Berry and colleagues (2016) reported that 30% of the full-sibs within a given litter were sired by 2 different rams; of the 137 sets of genotyped triplets in the study, 53% were sired by more than 1 ram. Unless the breeds of rams used were distinctly different with only 1 ram per breed, then sire parentage could not be resolved without resorting to genotyping the animals. Relatively recent estimates of parent-to-offspring parentage errors vary from 7.6% to 10.0% in sheep,[6] from 10.00% to 13.28% in cattle,[5,7,8] and from 8.4% to 14.6% in goats.[9] Nonetheless, the impact of parentage errors on an animal's estimate of genetic merit diminishes as the animal accumulates more (recorded) progeny with the impact deteriorating faster for higher heritability traits.[5] Where no parentage is known, then an ungenotyped newborn is typically assigned the breed average estimate of genetic merit.

The originally deployed genomic technology of microsatellites was really only useful for either confirming or excluding purported parentage. Additionally, it was feasible to investigate possible matches to a selection of other candidate parents upon request. SNP technology as a means of parentage testing officially started to replace microsatellite technology in cattle in 2012 based on the recommendation of the International Society of Animal Genetics. The International Society of Animal Genetics assumed responsibility for compiling a list of 100 to 200 internationally accepted SNPs for parentage verification. However, this panel size was not sufficient for parentage discovery. Furthermore, the fact that not all animals were genotyped meant that full parentage discovery was not feasible unless the genotypes of the parents were also accessible. Because of the ever-reducing cost of genotyping animals for circa 50,000 SNPs, more cattle populations (and a growing number of sheep populations) in developed countries are moving away from genotyping animals for just hundreds of SNPs but instead, opting to genotype animals for circa 50,000 SNPs which is very powerful for parentage discovery (assuming the parents are genotyped and those genotypes are accessible). If a country decides to embark on a national genotyping scheme, then biological samples from some of the parents may no longer be available for genotyping. However, it is possible, based on the genotypes of progeny (and also mates if available) to construct, *in silico*, the genotype of the parent(s).[10]

If entire populations are genotyped, then parentage discovery is certainly possible. However, once an entire population is genotyped, then the usefulness of actually knowing the parentage for breeding purposes diminishes. Genetic evaluations using dense genotypes can construct the pairwise relationships among individuals which are needed for genetic evaluations solely from genomic data without the need for any ancestral data. Furthermore, genomic information can provide far more accurate estimates of inbreeding of an individual or coancestry between individuals, than ancestral information ever can. This is because of the random inheritance of parental genotypes by offspring. Using a large population of both sheep and cattle, Kenny and colleagues (2023)[11] explored the genomic relationship among full-sib pairs. The mean genomic relationship between full-sibs born to unrelated, non-inbred parents matched the expectation of 0.50 but the standard deviation was 0.04. The extent of inbreeding of the parents, as well as their relationship also impacted the genomic relationship between full-sibs. Hence, recorded ancestry can only provide an estimate of the expected relationships between individuals in a population; the actual relationships can vary from this expectation and can only be determined through genotyping. More accurate estimates of the relationships among animals are important, given that it is a crucial component in genetic evaluations but knowing inter-animal relationships is also important for providing mating advice.

Traceability

Not only is traceability central to providing reassurance to consumers on the provenance of a sample, but traceability is also important in cases of lost animals or resolving disputes of alleged animal theft. Having an entire population genotyped for circa 50,000 SNPs provides excellent resolution in being able to match a taken sample to the correct individual. If accompanied by a national animal movement monitoring system as exists in European Union (EU) countries, then full traceability of animals and (most) meat products can be an excellent point of differentiation when trying to maintain or grow market share in the global meat market. Assuming the average of the least frequent variant of 1000 SNPs is 0.10, then the probability that 2 unrelated animals have an identical genotype is 9.3×10^{-193}.

Genes, Mutations, or Chromosomal Abnormalities of Major Effect

The field of quantitative genetics is underpinned by the infinitesimal model which, for quantitative traits, assumes an infinitely large number of DNA variants each having an infinitely small effect. While this assumption in genetic evaluation statistical models has certainly delivered genetic gain, DNA variants with large effects are known to exist—a good example is the nt821 mutation in the myostatin gene of cattle leading to a muscle hypertrophy phenotype, commonly known as double-muscling.[12] DNA variants have also been identified to cause differences in discrete traits like polledness[13] as well as congenital defects.[14]

While knowing the genotype of an individual for variants of major effect is useful when deciding the eventual fate of that animal (ie, for slaughter or as a parent of the next generation), having a national genotyping program enables the monitoring of trends in frequency of such variants in the population over time and, where warranted, prompts any national remedial action. Such corrective action at a national level could include the purging of undesirable variants; an example of such was the push to reduce or eradicate the frequency of scrapie-susceptible variants in sheep[15] or complex vertebral malformation in cattle.[16] Having a compulsory national genotyping strategy, accompanied by full disclosure of the resulting called genotypes, ensures transparency in the carrier status of animals. After all, you do not know you have something unless you test for it.

Genotyping all individuals, if accompanied by a centralised recording of any abnormal animal features, also facilitates the (rapid) detection of DNA variants contributing to large phenotypic differences; veterinarians and clinicians, as well as other professionals, including producers, have a role in recording such information to aid detection—information on, for example, the true frequency of the variant as well as the extent of population-wide segregation helps inform the likely mode of inheritance which, in turn, guides the investigative pathway. Genotyping dead animals, including stillborn animals, is also crucial. Even in the absence of phenotypic data, having access to a large population of genotyped animals also enables the detection of regions of the genome harboring lethal genetic variants. Lethal recessive genetic variants may be detected by comparing stretches of DNA (called haplotypes) that are common in a population but never (or rarely) appear in the homozygous state of live animals; VanRaden et al. (2001)[14] successfully used this approach in dairy cattle to detect 5 recessive defects in Holsteins, Jerseys, and Brown Swiss cows.

Therefore, a national genotyping scheme provides a realistic representation of the extent to which genes of major effect, including those conferring lethality, are segregating in a population. Crucially, because all animals are genotyped, it is not possible to conceal the carrier status of breeding animals at sales. It is important, however, that defects are centrally recorded and no shame is associated with owning such animals.

Spontaneous (ie, *de novo*) mutations constantly occur between generations; most are isolated cases, but even if they are of low frequency in a geographic location (eg, among a veterinarian's clients), having a national estimate of the frequency and the affected family lines can contribute to the appropriate management strategy.

Genomic Evaluations

Genome-enabled genomic evaluations, often simply called "genomic selection"[17] in the modern context, utilise genotypes from tens of thousands of SNP genotypes per individual to estimate its genetic merit. The high-level approach to genomic evaluations is similar to that of any prediction model; a calibration dataset exists of individuals with a series of outcome variables (eg, phenotypes like milk yield or growth rate) accompanied by a set of predictor variables which, in genomic selection, comprise approximately 50,000 features (ie, SNPs). A range of different algorithms and approaches to genomic evaluations have been described at length elsewhere[18] all to estimate the association effect between each of the model features (ie, SNP) and the outcome variable. These estimated SNP effects can then be applied to the genotype of a (newborn) individual and its genetic merit estimated. In reality, the approaches now implemented are more complex than this with many populations now transitioning to what is termed a "1-step approach"[19]; in 1-step genomic evaluations, all predictions are undertaken in 1 step, combining the pairwise animal relationships estimated from solely genomic data along with the relationships (among ungenotyped individuals) from recorded ancestry. Irrespective of the approach taken, the greater the number of phenotyped and genotyped individuals in the calibration population, the greater the accuracy of prediction; the strength of this relationship is influenced by several factors such as the accuracy of the estimate of genetic merit of the phenotyped animals but also the (genomic) relationship between the calibration dataset and the population where the predictions will be employed. The way in which the accuracy of genomic predictions changes with the size of the reference population for different trait heritabilities is illustrated in **Fig. 1**.[20] Clearly, a benefit exists of a national genomic scheme

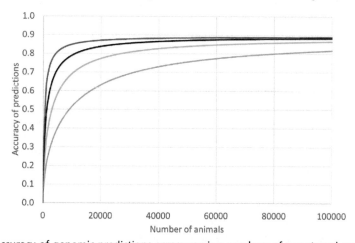

Fig. 1. Accuracy of genomic predictions across varying numbers of genotyped and phenotyped animals in a calibration dataset assuming a trait heritability of 0.05 (*blue line*), 0.15 (*green line*), 0.35 (*black line*), and 0.90 (*red line*) based on 1000 effective chromosome segments and where the genetic markers explain 80% of the genetic variance. (Daetwyler HD, Villanueva B, Woolliams JA, Accuracy of predicting the genetic risk of disease using a genome-wide approach. PLoS ONE 2008; 3: e3395.)

(where phenotypes already exist) in improving the accuracy of selection, especially for low heritability traits. However, the benefit eventually reaches a plateau.

Genetic gain per year can be summarized as[21]:

$$\text{Annual genetic gain} = \frac{\text{Selection intensity} \bullet \text{Accuracy of selection} \bullet \text{Genetic variabililty}}{\text{Generation interval}}$$

Hence, all else being equal, by being able to achieve a higher accuracy of selection, then genetic gain should accelerate. Moreover, because a genotype is available at birth, then the denominator term of the generation interval (ie, the average age of the animal when its progeny, who in turn also become parents, are born) can also be shortened, thus accelerating genetic gain even further. In fact, it is possible to genotype embryos[22] and thus, when coupled with advanced reproductive technologies like ovum pick up, the limiting factor of sexual maturity in females can be negated. Having the entire population genotyped also offers the potential to increase the selection intensity, again delivering step changes in genetic gain. While the accumulation of inbreeding in a functioning breeding program is always a concern, approaches such as optimal contribution theory[23] exist to help minimize this accumulation over time. In fact, genomic information can actually help reduce the rate of inbreeding accumulation, and having the whole population genotyped enables the detection of outcross individuals.

Precision Management

Although (accurate) prediction of genetic merit is important for delivering genetic gain, accurate predictions of genetic merit can, especially in the cases of high heritability traits, translate to relatively accurate predictions of phenotypic merit. Having a good estimate of expected phenotypic performance is important for identifying mature animals for purchasing or culling[24,25] but also for identifying younger animals for purchasing for meat production.[26] With a growing popularity of beef-on-dairy matings, the extent of integration between the dairy and beef sectors is strengthening. Most dairy farmers offload their surplus progeny at a very young age, a time when it can be difficult to gauge the expected carcass and feed efficiency potential of the animal. Although knowing the breed of the calf can help guide these predictions, considerable within-breed variability in a whole plethora of traits exist. Hence, having a genomic prediction of genetic merit for traits like growth, carcass merit, and feed intake could be very useful and if included in a national genomic testing scheme, then every animal could have such predictions. Growth, carcass, and feed intake traits in ruminants are moderate to highly heritable[27–29] implying that differences in genetic merit will, on average, be reflected in eventual phenotypic differences. The predictions of merit for individual traits could be combined into an index per animal where each trait is appropriately weighted[26] to aid in the selection process.

Having access to all the information from a genotype can help decide on the eventual fate of that animal; this is particularly so if the animal is genotyped at birth. If, for example, in an extreme case, the individual is found to have X-chromosomal monosomy (ie, Turners syndrome which is a case where the female has only 1 X chromosome) then she will be infertile; the ability to detect aneuploidy from SNP chip data has been demonstrated in cattle[30] and sheep.[31] Similarly, lambs with a copy of FecX^I and a copy of FecX^H mutations are infertile[32] as are lambs with 1 copy of FecX^G and FecX^B.[33] In these situations, the conclusion is obvious—there is no point in retaining the animal for breeding purposes so it should enter the production cycle for meat production. While genotyping just a herd or flock is sufficient to help make these decisions, and a national genotyping program is not required, a national genotyping program can provide the data necessary to identify new variants or abnormalities associated with sterility. A notable example of this was the detection of Swyer syndrome in the Irish cattle population. Typical females have 2 X chromosomes while a typical male has 1 X chromosome and 1 Y chromosome. Berry and colleagues (2023) described the detection of cattle with the Swyer condition in Ireland; a national genotyping strategy was launched to genotype females where farmers were financially incentivized to submit biological samples from females. Sex determination algorithms based on the presence of genotypes on the Y chromosome returned predictions of males from repeated samples of animals that were phenotypically females. On closer examination of the genomic sequence of the animals, these animals were indeed affected by Sywers syndrome and a test was developed to identify a large proportion of them based on the absence of the SRY gene.

Animal DNA is present in leukocytes (ie, white blood cells) which make up the majority of the reported somatic cell count values from milk testing. Milk with high numbers of somatic cells is often penalized financially and therefore identifying (and treating or culling) high cell count lactating animals is important to reduce the overall cell count of the farm's bulk milk. The milk from individual animals is often sampled on some farms, every 4 to 8 weeks, where the somatic cell count is estimated usually through flow cytometry. However, milk somatic cell count for individual animals can rise rapidly and thus may go undetected until the next individual animal milk test. Furthermore, not all farms participate in such milk testing strategies. However, bulk milk samples are usually taken from every collection of the milk. If the entire population of lactating animals contributing to the bulk milk is genotyped, then comparing the frequency of one of the alleles per SNP from the genotyped DNA extracted from the somatic cells in the bulk milk sample with that of the individual animals can identify the individuals with high somatic cell count. Individual animal milk recording should still be used to determine the milk yield and milk composition per animal, but these are generally very repeatable so records every 4 to 8 weeks should suffice to generate a good lactation average estimate. The approach of phenotyping the somatic cell count of genotyped individuals from the genotype of a bulk milk sample is now commercially available.

Homogeneity in a population often facilitates ease of management. Hence, producers might favor sires who generate more homogenous progeny; in contrast, breeders may actually seek sires who generate more heterogenous progeny, thereby increasing the probability of generating a genetically elite individual. Using the genotype of a sire coupled with an estimate of the effect of each SNP for a range of traits, it is possible to calculate the expected gametic variance of that sire[34] which should translate to differences in the heterogeneity of the progeny.[35] This strategy can be used to generate a more homogenous group of offspring. With a national genomic testing program, both genetic merit and expected heterogeneity of the genome can be determined for each animal. In a situation with more than 1 genetically elite animal of similar total merit, then the animal generating more homogenous progeny might be selected.

A developing approach is to use animal-side genome sequencing to not only rapidly determine the genotype of the animal itself but also non-host species. Early advancements in this approach, using Oxford Nanopore technology in beef cattle with the ability to detect pathogens associated with bovine respiratory disease, have been recently discussed.[36] At a national level, having such a system, albeit at just 1 point in time, could have considerable bearings on the use of vaccination for prevention of spread but also on the use of therapeutic treatment; this has obvious economic benefits but also reduces the pressure on the development of antimicrobial resistance. Furthermore, knowing the expected genetic predisposition of an animal to different attributes could alter the threshold governing when action should be taken. For example, the action taken, or indeed the treatment, for the same milk somatic cell count in lactating animals with different genetic predispositions to (sub-clinical) mastitis may differ. Similarly, interventions may be undertaken earlier post-partum in cows with a greater genetic susceptibility to anoestrus.

CHALLENGES TO IMPLEMENTATION OF A NATIONAL GENOTYPING STRATEGY

Fundamentally, industry segmentation creates a substantial barrier to a national genotyping (and associated phenotyping) initiative. The willingness to share data among sectors to improve the efficiency of an industry and farm-level decision-making requires a paradigm shift in many industries and a recognition of the value of genetic/genomic data to downstream management and marketing decisions and the value of non-seedstock data garnered to improve genetic gain. Consequently, for a national genotyping strategy to be successful, there must be a concerted buy-in and support for the initiative from all actors along the food production chain. One obvious barrier to the implementation of a national genotyping plan is the associated financial cost. Cost is not simply that associated with the genotyping platform itself but also the entire infrastructure and resources required for the efficient and effective operation of such an initiative. This includes the necessary laboratory infrastructure but also the computing hardware and software to enable data storage and analysis, as well as an effective traceability system to ensure stakeholders are always up-to-date on where in the pipeline a sample is. A menu of different funding models exists for such a large initiative with the optimal choice probably being a combination of the different options. Options include as follows:

- Exchequer and/or non-exchequer funding justified through improved efficiency of production and potentially reduced environmental footprint.
- Primary producer pays assuming a return on investment exists with the mode of deployment including either a single levy (such as at birth when registering an animal or at slaughter) or at different transactions throughout the animal's life.
- Industry itself (eg, milk and meat processors or livestock auctions).
- End consumer pays directly on a per unit of product purchased.

An additional barrier to implementation is the actual infrastructure and system of animal identification and traceability in the country. Ideally, all animals should have a unique national identification which remains with the animal throughout its life. All associated data relating to that animal should be linked to this identification and ideally accessible to all owners of the animal or its products (which includes processors). Having all these data accessible through a single, (independent) third-party, broker is helpful—this may not require all the data to be stored centrally but ideally pointers available from the brokerage infrastructure to the different databases facilitating rapid data retrieval. Encapsulated within this infrastructure requirement are the concerns associated with data privacy and security. Clear rules must be in place for data usage and state-of-the-art cybersecurity must be observed.

Sufficient resources also need to exist to clearly explain what can (and cannot) be done with the data and resulting information. This includes how the information generated from the genomic (and accompanying data) can be used to help different actors in the food chain improve their decision-making.

SUMMARY

Genomic information can provide a myriad of information to producers[4] including

- Reconciling parentage,
- Enabling traceability,
- Identifying carries of major genes including congenital defects as well as determining the change in their frequency in a population over time,
- Karyotyping,
- Quantifying breed composition,
- Determining animal gender,
- Providing information for more astute mating advice,
- Enabling greater precision in herd/flock management,
- Facilitating more accurate genomic evaluations for a range of different traits,

With the current state-of-the-art, where individuals are genotyped for circa 50,000 SNPs, sufficient information is generated to deliver these benefits from just a single biological sample. Being able to acquire that biological sample for genotyping at the time of birth, ideally where the sample can also be leveraged for other uses (eg, disease detection), further reduces the costs. All these contribute to a strong justification for a national genomic testing program, the greatest of which is an acceleration of genetic gain through greater accuracy of selection, as well as a potentially greater selection intensity and reduced generation interval. While genetic gain is often measured in monetary terms, most breeding goals are improving the environmental footprint of ruminant production systems; hence, national genotyping strategies can also potentially accelerate the reduction in the environmental footprint of the population.

CLINICS CARE POINTS

- Estimates of genetic merit of individuals are simply that—they are estimates. The confidence in those estimates is reflected by their stated accuracy or reliability metrics which is greater in genomically evaluated animals.
- Just because a dam and sire are genetically elite, it does not necessarily mean all the offspring will be.
- Litters of multiple individuals may be from multiple sires; this is common in mob-mated polyovulatory species.
- Knowing the carrier status of major genes or karyotypes of individual animals can help inform decisions on the fate of the animal as well as inform candidate matings.
- If a population is fully genotyped, the recorded ancestral information is not needed for genetic evaluations or for designing mating plans.
- Biological samples of animals with uncommon features along with both their parents should be taken for genomic analysis; samples from unaffected siblings should also be retained.

DISCLOSURE

The authors have no conflict of interest.

REFERENCES

1. Villanueva B, Pong-Wong R, Fernández J, et al. Benefits from marker-assisted selection under an additive polygenic genetic model. J Anim Sci 2005;83:1747–52.

2. Van Eenennaam AL, Li J, Thallman RM, et al. Validation of commercial DNA tests for quantitative beef quality traits. J Anim Sci 2007;85:891–900.

3. Zhao S, Jing W, Samuels DC, et al. Strategies for processing and quality control of Illumina genotyping arrays. Brief Bioinform 2018;19:765–75.

4. Berry D.P. and Spangler M.L. Practical applications of genomic information in livestock, *Animal*, 2023, Submitted. Paper no. 100996.

5. Visscher PM, Woolliams JA, Smith D, et al. Estimation of pedigree errors in the UK dairy population using microsatellite markers and the impact on selection. J Dairy Sci 2002;85:2368–75.

6. Berry DP, O'Brien A, Wall E, et al. Inter-and intra-reproducibility of genotypes from sheep technical replicates on Illumina and Affymetrix platforms. Gen, Sel Evol 2016;48:86–94.

7. Purfield DC, McClure M, Berry DP. Justification for setting the individual animal genotype call rate threshold at eighty-five percent. J Anim Sci 2016;94:4558–69.

8. Řehout V, Hradecká E, Čítek E. Evaluation of parentage testing in the Czech population of Holstein cattle. Czech J Anim Sci 2006;51:503–9.

9. Bolormaa S, Ruvinsky A, Walkden-Brown S, et al. DNA-based parentage verification in two Australian goat herds. Small Rumin Res 2008;80:95–100.

10. Berry DP, McParland S, Kearney JF, et al. Imputation of ungenotyped parental genotypes in dairy and beef cattle from progeny genotypes. Animal 2014;8:895–903.

11. Kenny D, Berry DP, Pabiou T, et al. Variation in the proportion of the segregating genome shared between full-sibling cattle and sheep. Genet Sel Evol 2023;55:1–7.

12. McPherron AC, Lee SJ. Double muscling in cattle due to mutations in the myostatin gene. Proc Natl Acad Sci U S A 1997;94:12457–61.

13. Medugorac I, Seichter D, Graf A, et al. Bovine polledness – an autosomal dominant trait with allelic heterogeneity. PLoS One 2012;7.

14. VanRaden PM, Olson KM, Null DJ, et al. Harmful recessive effects on fertility detected by absence of homozygous haplotypes. J Dairy Sci 2011;94:6153–61.

15. Gubbins S, Webb CR. Simulation of the options for a national control programme to eradicate scrapie from Great Britain. Prev Vet Med 2005;69:175–87.

16. Rusc A, Hering D, Puckowska P, et al. Screening of Polish Holstein-Friesian bulls towards eradication of Complex Vertebral Malformation (CVM) carriers. Pol J Vet Sci 2013;16:579–81.

17. Meuwissen THE, Hayes BJ, Goddard ME. Prediction of total genetic value using genome-wide dense marker maps. Genetics 2001;157:1819–29.

18. Legarra A, Christensen OF, Aguilar I, et al. Single Step, a general approach for genomic selection. Livest Sci 2014;166:54–65.

19. Lourenco D, Legarra A, Tsuruta S, et al. Single-step genomic evaluations from theory to practice: using SNP chips and sequence data in BLUPF90. Genesis 2020;11:790. https://doi.org/10.3390/genes11070790.

20. Daetwyler HD, Villanueva B, Woolliams JA. Accuracy of predicting the genetic risk of disease using a genome-wide approach. PLoS One 2008;3:e3395.

21. Rendel J, Robertson A. Estimation of genetic gain in milk yield by selection in a closed herd of dairy cattle. J Genet 1950;50:1–8.

22. Mullaart E, Wells D. Embryo Biopsies for Genomic Selection. In: Niemann H, Wrenzycki C, editors. Animal Biotechnology, 2. Cham: Springer; 2018. https://doi.org/10.1007/978-3-319-92348-2_5.

23. Woolliams JA, Berg P, Dagnachew BS, et al. Genetic contributions and their optimization. J Anim Breed Genet 2015;132:89–99.

24. Kelleher MM, Amer PR, Shalloo L, et al. Development of an index to rank dairy females on expected lifetime profit. J Dairy Sci 2015;98:4225–39.
25. Dunne FL, Berry DP, Kelleher MM, et al. An index framework founded on the future profit potential of female beef cattle to aid the identification of candidates for culling. J Anim Sci 2020a;98:1–14.
26. Dunne FL, Evans RD, Kelleher MM, et al. Formulation of a decision support tool incorporating both genetic and non-genetic effects to rank young growing cattle on expected market value. Animal 2020b;15:100077.
27. Schiermiester LN, Thallman RM, Kuehn LA, et al. 2015. Estimation of breed-specific heterosis effects for birth, weaning, and yearling weight in cattle. J Anim Sci 2015;93:46–52.
28. McHugh N, Pabiou T, McDermott K, et al. Genetic (co)variance components for slaughter traits in a multi-breed sheep population. Animal 2023;17:100883.
29. Torres-Vázquez JA, Spangler ML. Genetic parameters for docility, weaning weight, yearling weight, and intramuscular fat percentage in Hereford cattle. J Anim Sci 2016;94:21–7.
30. Berry DP, Wolfe A, O'Donovan J, et al. Characterization of an X-chromosomal non-mosaic monosomy (59, X0) dairy heifer detected using routinely available single nucleotide polymorphism genotype data. J Anim Sci 2017;95:1042–9.
31. Berry DP, O'Brien A, O'Donovan J, et al. Aneuploidy in dizygotic twin sheep detected using genome-wide single nucleotide polymorphism data from two commonly used commercial vendors. Animal 2018;12:2462–9.
32. Davis GH, Dodds KG, Wheeler R, et al. Evidence that an imprinted gene on the X chromosome increases ovulation rate in sheep. Biol Reprod 2001;64:216–21.
33. Hanrahan JP, Gregan SM, Mulsant P, et al. Mutations in the genes for oocyte derived growth factors GDF9 and BMP15 are associated with both increased ovulation rate and sterility in Cambridge and Belclare sheep (Ovis aries). Biol Reprod 2004;70:900–9.
34. Santos DJA, Cole JB, Lawlor Jr TJ, et al. Variance of gametic diversity and its application in selection programs. J Dairy Sci 2019;102:5279–94.
35. Hozé C, Baur A, Fritz S, et al. Prediction of gametic variance and its use in bovine breeding programs. Proceedings of 12th World Congress on Genetics Applied to Livestock Production, 2022, (WCGALP); Rotterdam The Netherlands, 3364.
36. Lamb H.J., On-farm genotyping to accelerate genetic gain in Australia's northern beef industry, A thesis submitted for the degree of Doctor of Philosophy at The University of Queensland, 2023. PhD thesis.

Advancing Dairy and Beef Genetics Through Genomic Technologies

Priyanka Banerjee, PhD, Wellison J.S. Diniz, PhD*

KEYWORDS

- Beef genomics • Dairy genomics • Genomic selection • Selective breeding
- Sustainability

KEY POINTS

- The US beef and dairy industries have made remarkable advances in sustainability.
- Selective breeding of animals with high genetic value has significantly enhanced productivity.
- To address the demand for sustainable production systems, there is a shift toward selecting for efficiency and fitness traits.
- Genome editing, high-throughput phenotyping, and other emerging technologies offer promising avenues for further genetic progress in cattle breeding.

INTRODUCTION

The livestock industry is a key player in addressing the current challenges facing global food security.[1] Challenges are not only related to the forecasted increased demand for animal-derived food products due to the growing population, they also encompass the need for more sustainable production systems. Furthermore, climate change and the availability of natural resources, including water and arable land, will affect agricultural production when the demand for food products is expected to increase by 70% by 2050.[1–3] Addressing these challenges requires several actions, which include improving animal productivity and efficiency. In this direction, the US beef and dairy industries have progressed toward sustainable practices, using fewer natural resources and increasing productivity.[4,5]

In addition to technological and management practices, selective breeding of animals with high genetic value has significantly enhanced productivity. For instance, beef and milk production have seen marked increases over the last decades despite a significant reduction in the size of the herd.[4–6] This progress relied on statistical

Department of Animal Sciences, Auburn University, Auburn, AL 36849, USA
* Corresponding author.
E-mail address: wzd0027@auburn.edu

Vet Clin Food Anim 40 (2024) 447–458
https://doi.org/10.1016/j.cvfa.2024.05.009   **vetfood.theclinics.com**
0749-0720/24/© 2024 Elsevier Inc. All rights are reserved, including those for text and data mining, AI training, and similar technologies.

methods using best linear unbiased prediction models, which integrate phenotypic measurements of economically important traits and pedigree information to estimate breeding values (EBVs).[7] Despite its success, genetic progress has limitations, including phenotype availability and costs, timely selection of breeding animals, and the complex nature of quantitative traits.[7,8] To overcome these challenges, different methods have been implemented.[8]

Technological innovations, such as DNA sequencing and genotyping and high-throughput phenotyping, have provided new avenues to address the pressure for efficiency and sustainability that the cattle industry currently faces. Recently, gene editing has created promising opportunities and has been added to the breeding toolbox. Thus, the synergistic use of these technologies has the potential to provide a better understanding of the structure and function of the genome and their interplay with the environment.[9,10] Therefore, in this review, the authors explore recent developments in genomics applied to beef and dairy breeding, highlighting opportunities and challenges for production and health improvement.

Genomic Research in Beef and Dairy Cattle

Cattle production is a critical component of the US economy[6] and accounted for USD 86.1 billion in total farm receipts in 2022.[11] Despite advances, intrinsic differences in the dairy and beef industries have led to varying rates of genetic gain. Common to both has been the selective breeding for production-related traits such as early growth and milk production.[12,13] However, intensive selection has resulted in unfavorable responses in reproductive and health-related traits,[14] which were not previously included in the breeding programs. Additionally, with the current demands for sustainable and resilient production systems, there is a need to select for novel traits, such as efficiency, longevity, health, fertility, temperament, and conformation.[14,15]

The advances in next-generation sequencing and the availability of the cattle genome have enhanced our understanding about the genetic architecture of complex traits and opened new possibilities for animal genomics research and tools to genetically improve cattle. Traditional methods and applications of molecular-based approaches have been reviewed.[8,16] Likewise, Rolf and colleagues[17] have discussed the unique challenges of the beef industry in translating and using genomic tools. Almost a decade after these reviews, progress has been made in deploying genomic selection (GS) in the beef industry. GS is based on genomic estimated breeding values (GEBVs) that are estimated by calculating single nucleotide polymorphisms (SNP) effects from a reference population. The accuracy of GEBVs is contingent upon the size of the reference population, the heritability of the trait, and the degree of relationships between the selection candidates and the reference population.[7,13,18] The partnership between breed associations and biotechnology companies has resulted in the development of commercial tests that go beyond parentage tests and the identification of carriers of deleterious mutations. Currently, companies such as Zoetis and Neogen have commercially available genetic tests that evaluate genetic merit through economic indexes or genomic-enhanced expected progeny differences or predicted transmitting abilities (PTAs) for purebred and crossbred cattle.

Advances in the Dairy Industry

The genetic progress in the dairy industry since the implementation of GS showcases its benefits over traditional selection, mainly for lowly heritable traits such as somatic cell score (SCS), daughter pregnancy rate, and productive life.[19] This is due to the increased accuracy and reduced generation interval.[19,20] For Holstein bulls born in 2017 and cows born in 2019, generation intervals of 2.2, 3.9, 2.2, and 3.1 years were reported for sire of bulls, sires of cows, dams of bulls, and dams of cows, respectively.[21] The decline was also reported for sires of the Brown Swiss and Jersey breeds.[21] Since the implementation of GS, increases in cow profitability measured through Net Merit (NM$) were also reported[20] (**Fig. 1**). The NM$ index accounts for more than 40 traits and is the primary dairy genetic selection index in the United States.[13] However, the priorities of these traits within the index have changed overtime from yield to fitness traits.[13,22]

Decreased fertility has been one of the challenges that both the beef and dairy industries face. As shown in **Fig. 1**, there was a continuous decrease in both daughter pregnancy and cow conception rates. Genetic progress for fertility-related traits has been reported since their inclusion in breeding programs combined with GS. While

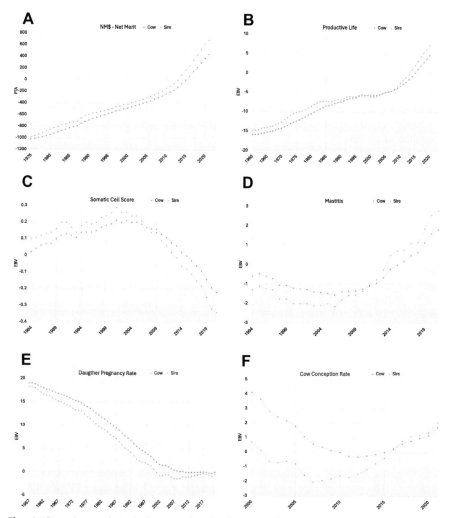

Fig. 1. Genetic trends in indexes and traits for US Holstein cows and sires by birth year (December 2023, evaluation). Based on (*A*) NM$, (*B*) productive life, (*C*) somatic cell score, (*D*) mastitis, (*E*) daughter pregnancy rate, and (*F*) cow conception rate. (*Data from* The Council on Dairy Cattle Breeding [https://webconnect.uscdcb.com/#/summary-stats/genetic-trend].)

the major focus has been on understanding the genetic basis of female fertility,[23,24] it has been shown that males are key players in pregnancy success.[25,26] Currently, the national genetic evaluations of dairy breeds led by the Council on Dairy Cattle Breeding (CDCB) have included daughter pregnancy rate, cow conception rate, calving to first insemination, gestation length, and early first calving.[27] The service–sire relative conception rate is used to measure male fertility.[27] Novel traits have also been proposed to address the low heritability of traditional fertility measures, including mid-infrared spectroscopy (MFERT) and reproductive tract size and position score (SPS).[28,29] The findings reported from these studies were exploratory due to the limited sample size. However, the authors highlighted that as the number of records for MFERT increases, so will the accuracy of prediction.[30] Similarly, SPS has the potential to be used as an indicator trait for fertility as it was favorably genetically correlated with nonreturn rate at 56 days and first service to conception.[29]

Mastitis is the most prominent and economically significant disease in the dairy industry. Indirect measurement of mastitis resistance was based on low SCS.[31] However, since 2018, mastitis has been included among other health-related traits in genetic evaluations.[27] **Fig. 1** shows a decrease in the EBVs for SCS and an increase in the EBVs for mastitis. According to the CDCB, animals with PTA SCS less than 3.0 are expected to transmit favorable udder health, while increased EBVs for mastitis represent the expected resistance of an animal's offspring to clinical mastitis.[32] These traits are genetically negatively correlated (r = − 0.68), indicating SCS decreases as resistance to mastitis increases.[33]

Selection for novel traits, such as immune response (IR), has also shown promising results, as dairy cows with higher IR showed increased resistance to mastitis.[34] In Holstein cows, IR measured as antibody-mediated immune responses (AMIR) and cell-mediated immune responses (CMIR) were reported as moderately heritable.[34] Likewise, a genome-wide association study of cows classified as high or low for AMIR or CMIR showed significant variation in SNP profiles, with significant markers overrepresented in chromosome 23.[35] Interestingly, IR was genetically positively correlated with the number of services and first service to conception.[34] A large-scale study of disease incidence for daughters of sires with high immunity in commercial dairy herds found significantly reduced incidences of mastitis, lameness, mortality, and overall disease for progeny sired by bulls with high EBVs for IR.[36]

Breeding for efficient cows has also gained interest not only from a producer's point of view to increase profitability but also as a tool to address the current environmental demands for sustainability. Feed-efficient animals would eat less feed while maintaining similar production to their herd mates.[37] Additionally, studies have shown that feed-efficient cows would emit less methane.[38] Residual feed intake (RFI) is currently the main metric used to measure feed efficiency, which is based on the difference between the actual and expected dry matter intake after adjusting for metabolic body weight and level of production.[39] The heritability estimate of RFI was 0.24 ($\pm$0.02), based on the genomic evaluation of US Holstein cows.[37] Inclusion of feed intake data in the NM\$ selection index can have a large impact on profitability.[40] The CDCB has developed the feed saved trait (FSAV) as a measure of efficiency by combining the benefits of reduced RFI and smaller body weight composite.[40,41] Currently, FSAV accounts for +13.2% of the weight in the NM\$ index.[22] While the inclusion of feed efficiency-related traits shows promising results, the amount of data available is still a limiting factor. To overcome this, it has been suggested not only to increase data collection but also to share data across multiple countries. Bolormaa and colleagues[42] reported that combining data from international partners can improve the accuracy of prediction for feed efficiency. An example of such an initiative is the Resilient Dairy Genome Project, in which 7 countries share feed efficiency-related data, including methane emission and RFI, to generate genomic tools to breed more resilient dairy cows.[43]

Advances in the Beef Industry

Genomic application in the beef industry is already underway, although at a low pace compared to the dairy industry. This is due to the several factors previously discussed by Berry and colleagues[44] and Rolf and colleagues.[17] Several of the challenges pointed out by these authors are being addressed, including the acceptance of this technology by producers and the number of animals genomically evaluated. A survey with beef producers in Tennessee regarding the adoption of genomic tests indicated that 74% of them were interested in using this technology to select replacement heifers and 56% for marketing cattle.[45]

A growing number of studies have explored the potential of genomics to understand the genetic factors involved with cow efficiency and sustainability.[46] Underlying traits are not only related to yield but also health, fertility, longevity, feed efficiency, and methane emission. Beef breed associations have embraced DNA tests as a tool for genetic evaluation and selection programs. Additionally, biotechnology companies such as Neogen and Zoetis have developed genomic tests to assist beef producers in their breeding decisions (**Table 1**). These companies are also partnering with breed associations to develop customized tests. For example, the GeneMax Advantage test has been designed for selecting and mating Angus-based replacement females and provides predictions for 17 maternal, feedlot, and carcass traits and 3 economic indexes.[47] Arisman and colleagues[48] evaluated the accuracy of the GeneMax advantage test in a commercial Angus herd and reported that the test accurately predicted the heifer's genetic merit. Opportunities have also been developed for feeder cattle marketed to feedlots, focusing on postweaning growth, feed efficiency, and carcass merit.

The American Angus Association has led the implementation of genomic evaluation in the United States.[44] For other breed associations, genomic evaluation was implemented through collaboration with the International Genetic Solutions to carry out a multi-breed evaluation, hosting a database with 20 million animals and over 300,000 genotypes.[49] Currently, over 1 million American Angus animals have been genotyped, and an increase in accuracy and a decrease in generation interval have already been reported.[50,51] The rates of genetic progress for growth (weaning weight) and carcass traits (carcass weight and ribeye area) have also benefited from GS.[50]

The National Cattle Evaluation Consortium has coordinated priorities for beef genetic evaluation in the United States.[52] Similarly, the Beef Improvement Federation has provided guidelines for Uniform Beef Improvement Programs and the traits to be recorded for genetic prediction.[53] This has been implemented through an inventory-based whole herd reporting system that encompasses the production of every cow and the performance of every calf raised through weaning for the year.[54] However, the genetic evaluations for the traits reported are variable according to the breeding association.[12] Common between them is the focus on growth and carcass traits. Recently, novel traits have been incorporated with a focus on longevity, fertility, and temperament.[55,56]

Other Omics Technologies and Opportunities

Remarkable progress has been achieved through the implementation of genomics in breeding decisions. However, alongside genomics, other technologies have been employed to understand the genome function and regulation that underlie

Table 1
Commercially available genomic tests for beef cattle

Company[a]	Tests	Market/Focus	Breeds	Traits
Zoetis®	INHERIT® Select[b]	Crossbred replacement females	Angus, Red Angus, South Devon, Hereford, Simmental, Gelbvieh, Limousin, and Charolais	19 traits and 5 economic indexes[57]
	INHERIT® Optimize and INHERIT® Market	Commercial feeder		Postweaning growth, feed efficiency, and carcass merit.
	GeneMax® Advantage™	Replacement heifers	Angus (75% or greater)	17 genomic trait scores for maternal, feedlot and carcass traits, and 3 economic indexes[47]
Neogen®	Igenity® Angus Gold	Replacement heifers	Angus (75% or greater)	Igenity Scores for 15 key maternal, performance, and carcass traits[58]
	Igenity® Beef	Crossbred commercial heifers and steers	Angus, Gelbvieh, Hereford, Limousin, Maine-Anjou, Red Angus, Shorthorn, Simmental	Igenity Scores for 17 key maternal, performance, and carcass traits as well as 3 indexes[59]
	Igenity® Envigor™	Crossbred cattle and select replacements	Angus, Brahman, Gelbvieh, Hereford, Limousin, Red Angus, Simmental, Wagyu, and many other breeds of cattle	Measure heterosis in crossbred cattle[60]
	Igenity® Feeder	Stocker, backgrounder, and feedlot	Angus, Gelbvieh, Hereford, Limousin, Maine-Anjou, Red Angus, Shorthorn, Simmental	Igenity Terminal Index and Igenity DOF Index[61]
	Igenity® BeefxDairy	Beef on dairy calf performance	Beef breeds: Angus, Brahman, Gelbvieh, Hereford, Limousin, Red Angus, Shorthorn, Simmental, and Waygu, Dairy breeds: Holstein and Jersey	Average Daily Gain, Hot Carcass Weight, Marbling (IMF), Igenity Terminal Index[62]

[a] Mention of a trade name or commercial product does not constitute or imply its endorsement by the authors.
[b] Exclusively for females.

economically important traits. Studies in transcriptomics, proteomics, metabolomics, and epigenomics have shed light on functional changes between individuals under different treatments or management conditions. The study of the microbiome has enhanced our understanding of host genome–microbiome interactions. Improvements in accuracy have been reported by incorporating the microbiome information into genomic prediction models.[63,64] Recently, the opportunities for genome editing through the CRISPR-cas9 system have been a paradigm shift for genetic improvement. A few studies in livestock have showcased the potential of this system,[9] including the generation of a gene-edited calf with resistance to bovine viral diarrhea virus infection.[65] Further progress is expected as these technologies are integrated with assisted reproductive technologies.[9,51]

Translating functional results into field applications remains a challenge. The "USDA Blueprint for Improving Animal Production" emphasizes the need for an in-depth understanding of genome biology to empower GS.[10] The Functional Annotation of Animal Genomes project has also highlighted priorities to understand genome function and regulation and improvement of livestock animals.[66] Emerging opportunities are anticipated for using sensors in high-throughput phenotyping, breeding, and precise management.[67] Despite the vast amount of information, there is a need for statistical methods to effectively integrate and utilize these data for GS. Current approaches include intermediate omics features,[68] multilayer neural networks,[69] and machine learning.[70]

SUMMARY

In this review, we discussed the key role of genomic advancements in addressing challenges within the US cattle industry, such as the increasing demand for sustainable and efficient production systems. Additionally, we highlighted the use of GS leading to improved productivity and the selection of novel traits. Despite these advancements, challenges remain in the recording of novel phenotypes. Opportunities, however, are foreseen through the developments and use of sensor technologies for real-time animal monitoring.

CLINICS CARE POINTS

- Selective breeding powered by genomic tools has enabled the selection of novel traits and increased the rate of genetic progress, contributing to overall herd efficiency and profitability.

- The combination of molecular and reproductive technologies has maximized genetic gain in the livestock industry. The emerging use of gene editing technology offers promising opportunities to address cattle sustainability.

- Genomic tests are now available to multiple production sectors of the beef industry. Decreasing costs and understanding the benefits of GS have led to increased adoption of genomic selection by beef producers.

- Low heritable phenotypes, recording from extensively managed herds, and the availability of suitable data for genetic evaluation are still challenges for the beef industry.

DISCLOSURE

The authors declare no conflicts of interest.

FUNDING

This project was financially supported by the Agricultural Research Service, U.S. Department of Agriculture, under agreement no. 58-6010-1-005, and the Alabama Agricultural Experiment Station—Hatch program of the National Institute of Food and Agriculture, U.S. Department of Agriculture.

REFERENCES

1. Council NR. Critical role of animal science research in food security and sustainability. Washington, DC: The National Academies Press; 2015. https://doi.org/10.17226/19000.
2. FAO. Global agriculture towards 2050. In: High-level expert forum - how to feed the world in 2050. 2009. Rome: Available at: http://www.fao.org/fileadmin/templates/wsfs/docs/Issues_papers/HLEF2050_Global_Agriculture.pdf.
3. Rojas-Downing MM, Nejadhashemi AP, Harrigan T, et al. Climate change and livestock: Impacts, adaptation, and mitigation. Clim Risk Manag 2017;16:145–63. https://doi.org/10.1016/j.crm.2017.02.001.
4. Capper JL. The environmental impact of beef production in the United States: 1977 compared with 2007. J Anim Sci 2011;89(12):4249–61. https://doi.org/10.2527/JAS.2010-3784.
5. Capper JL, Cady RA, Bauman DE. The environmental impact of dairy production: 1944 compared with 20071. J Anim Sci 2009;87(6):2160–7. https://doi.org/10.2527/jas.2009-1781.
6. USDA. USDA ERS - Sector at a Glance. Available at: https://www.ers.usda.gov/topics/animal-products/cattle-beef/sector-at-a-glance/. 2023. https://www.ers.usda.gov/topics/animal-products/cattle-beef/sector-at-a-glance/. Accessed June 5, 2023.
7. Dekkers JCM. Application of Genomics Tools to Animal Breeding. Curr Genom 2012;13(3):207–12. https://doi.org/10.2174/138920212800543057.
8. Nayeri S, Sargolzaei M, Tulpan D. A review of traditional and machine learning methods applied to animal breeding. Anim Health Res Rev 2019;20(1):31–46. https://doi.org/10.1017/S1466252319000148.
9. Mueller ML, Van Eenennaam AL. Synergistic power of genomic selection, assisted reproductive technologies, and gene editing to drive genetic improvement of cattle. CABI Agric Biosci 2022;3(1):13. https://doi.org/10.1186/s43170-022-00080-z.
10. Rexroad C, Vallet J, Matukumalli LK, et al. Genome to Phenome: Improving Animal Health, Production, and Well-Being – A New USDA Blueprint for Animal Genome Research 2018–2027. Front Genet 2019;10:237. https://doi.org/10.3389/fgene.2019.00327.
11. USDA ERS. Usda ERS - 2022 U.S. animal and animal products cash receipts. USDA; 2023. Available at: https://www.ers.usda.gov/data-products/chart-gallery/gallery/chart-detail/?chartId=76949. [Accessed 14 February 2024].
12. Garrick DJ. The nature, scope and impact of genomic prediction in beef cattle in the United States. Genet Sel Evol 2011;43(1):17. https://doi.org/10.1186/1297-9686-43-17.
13. Van Eenennaam AL, Weigel KA, Young AE, et al. Applied animal genomics: results from the field. Annu Rev Anim Biosci 2013. https://doi.org/10.1146/annurev-animal-022513-114119.
14. Brito LF, Bedere N, Douhard F, et al. Review: Genetic selection of high-yielding dairy cattle toward sustainable farming systems in a rapidly changing world. Animal 2021;15:100292. https://doi.org/10.1016/j.animal.2021.100292.

15. Egger-Danner C, Cole JB, Pryce JE, et al. Invited review: overview of new traits and phenotyping strategies in dairy cattle with a focus on functional traits. Animal 2015;9(2):191–207. https://doi.org/10.1017/S1751731114002614.

16. Blasco A, Toro MA. A short critical history of the application of genomics to animal breeding. Livest Sci 2014;166(1):4–9. https://doi.org/10.1016/j.livsci.2014.03.015.

17. Rolf MM, Decker JE, McKay SD, et al. Genomics in the United States beef industry. Livest Sci 2014;166(1):84–93. https://doi.org/10.1016/j.livsci.2014.06.005.

18. Hayes BJ, Lewin HA, Goddard ME. The future of livestock breeding: genomic selection for efficiency, reduced emissions intensity, and adaptation. Trends Genet 2013;29(4):206–14. https://doi.org/10.1016/j.tig.2012.11.009.

19. García-Ruiz A, Cole JB, VanRaden PM, et al. Changes in genetic selection differentials and generation intervals in US Holstein dairy cattle as a result of genomic selection. Proc Natl Acad Sci USA 2016;113(28):E3995–4004. https://doi.org/10.1073/pnas.1519061113.

20. Wiggans GR, Cole JB, Hubbard SM, et al. Genomic selection in dairy cattle: The USDA experience. Annu Rev Anim Biosci 2017;5(1):309–27. https://doi.org/10.1146/annurev-animal-021815-111422.

21. Guinan FL, Wiggans GR, Norman HD, et al. Changes in genetic trends in US dairy cattle since the implementation of genomic selection. J Dairy Sci 2023;106(2):1110–29. https://doi.org/10.3168/jds.2022-22205.

22. Vanraden PM, Cole JB, Neupane M, et al. Net merit as a measure of lifetime profit: 2021 revision. AIP Res Rep NM$8 2021. Available at: http://go.usa.gov/xybuq. [Accessed 17 February 2024].

23. Ma L, Cole JB, Da Y, et al. Symposium review: Genetics, genome-wide association study, and genetic improvement of dairy fertility traits. J Dairy Sci 2019;102(4):3735–43. https://doi.org/10.3168/jds.2018-15269.

24. Spencer TE, Hansen PJ, Cole JB, et al. Genomic selection and reproductive efficiency in dairy cattle. In: Dairy cattle reproduction conference. Salt Lake City: the dairy cattle reproduction Council does. 2014. p. 16–31. Available at: https://s3.wp.wsu.edu/uploads/sites/2147/2015/03/Spencer-DCRC-Genomics-Fertility-20141.pdf.

25. Han Y, Peñagaricano F. Unravelling the genomic architecture of bull fertility in Holstein cattle. BMC Genet 2016;17(1):143. https://doi.org/10.1186/s12863-016-0454-6.

26. Taylor JF, Schnabel RD, Sutovsky P. Review: Genomics of bull fertility. Animal 2018;12(s1):s172–83. https://doi.org/10.1017/S1751731118000599.

27. Wiggans GR, Carrillo JA. Genomic selection in United States dairy cattle. Front Genet 2022;13:994466. https://doi.org/10.3389/FGENE.2022.994466/BIBTEX.

28. Van den Berg I, Stephen M, Ho PN, et al. New phenotypes for genetic improvement of fertility in dairy cows. In: Hermesch S, Dominik S, editors. *Breeding focus 2021 - improving reproduction*. Armidale, NSW, Australia: animal genetics and breeding unit. 2021. p. 187. Available at: http://agbu.une.edu.au. [Accessed 4 June 2022].

29. Martin AA, de Oliveira Jr G, Madureira AM, et al. Reproductive tract size and position score: Estimation of genetic parameters for a novel fertility trait in dairy cows. J Dairy Sci 2022;105:8189–98. https://doi.org/10.3168/jds.2021-21651.

30. van den Berg I, Ho PN, Haile-Mariam M, et al. Genetic parameters for mid-infrared spectroscopy–predicted fertility. JDS Commun 2021;2(6):361–5. https://doi.org/10.3168/jdsc.2021-0141.

31. Weigel KA, Shook GE. Genetic Selection for Mastitis Resistance. Vet Clin North Am Food Anim Pract 2018;34(3):457–72. https://doi.org/10.1016/j.cvfa.2018.07.001.

32. CDCB. Individual Traits - CDCB. 2024. Available at: https://uscdcb.com/individual-traits/. [Accessed 17 February 2024].

33. CDCB. Trait reference sheet - resistance to mastitis (MAST) 2018. https://doi.org/10.3168/jds.2017-13554.

34. Thompson-Crispi KA, Sewalem A, Miglior F, et al. Genetic parameters of adaptive immune response traits in Canadian Holsteins. J Dairy Sci 2012;95(1):401–9. https://doi.org/10.3168/jds.2011-4452.

35. Thompson-Crispi KA, Sargolzaei M, Ventura R, et al. A genome-wide association study of immune response traits in Canadian Holstein cattle. BMC Genom 2014; 15(1):1–10. https://doi.org/10.1186/1471-2164-15-559/FIGURES/6.

36. Larmer S, Mallard B. High immune response sires reduce disease incidence in North American large commercial dairy populations. Cattle Pract 2017;25:74–81.

37. Khanal P, Johnson J, Gouveia G, et al. Genomic evaluation of feed efficiency in US Holstein heifers. J Dairy Sci 2023;106(10):6986–94. https://doi.org/10.3168/JDS.2023-23258.

38. de Haas Y, Windig JJ, Calus MPL, et al. Genetic parameters for predicted methane production and potential for reducing enteric emissions through genomic selection. J Dairy Sci 2011;94(12):6122–34. https://doi.org/10.3168/jds.2011-4439.

39. Brito LF, Oliveira HR, Houlahan K, et al. Genetic mechanisms underlying feed utilization and implementation of genomic selection for improved feed efficiency in dairy cattle. In: Plaizier J, editor. Can J Anim Sci 2020;100(4):587–604. https://doi.org/10.1139/cjas-2019-0193.

40. Vanraden PM, O'connell JR, Connor EE, et al. Including Feed Intake Data from U.S. Holsteins in Genomic Prediction. Vol 11.; 2018:125. Available at: https://aipl.arsusda.gov/publish/other/2018/WCGALP2018_VanRaden.pdf.

41. CDCB. Trait reference sheet - Feed Saved (FSAV). 2020. Available at: https://uscdcb.com/wp-content/uploads/2020/11/CDCB-Reference-Sheet-Feed-Saved-12_2020.pdf. [Accessed 18 February 2024].

42. Bolormaa S, MacLeod IM, Khansefid M, et al. Sharing of either phenotypes or genetic variants can increase the accuracy of genomic prediction of feed efficiency. Genet Sel Evol 2022;54(1):1–17. https://doi.org/10.1186/S12711-022-00749-Z/TABLES/7.

43. van Staaveren N, Oliveira HR, Houlahan K, et al. The Resilient Dairy Genome Project – a general overview of methods and objectives related to feed efficiency and methane emissions. J Dairy Sci 2023. https://doi.org/10.3168/jds.2022-22951.

44. Berry DP, Garcia JF, Garrick DJ. Development and implementation of genomic predictions in beef cattle. Anim Front 2016;6(1):32–8. https://doi.org/10.2527/af.2016-0005.

45. DeLong KL, Jensen KL, Griffith AP, et al. Feeder cattle genomic tests: Analyzing cattle producer adoption decisions. J Agric Appl Econ Assoc 2023;2(2):334–49. https://doi.org/10.1002/jaa2.61.

46. Rowan TN. Invited Review: Genetic decision tools for increasing cow efficiency and sustainability in forage-based beef systems. Appl Anim Sci 2022;38(6):660–70. https://doi.org/10.15232/aas.2022-02306.

47. Zoetis. Implementing GENEMAX advantage. 2023. Available at: www.angus.org/agi. [Accessed 19 August 2023].

48. Arisman BC, Rowan TN, Thomas JM, et al. Evaluation of Zoetis GeneMax Advantage genomic predictions in commercial Bos taurus Angus cattle. Livest Sci 2023;274:105266. https://doi.org/10.1016/j.livsci.2023.105266.

49. IGS. Multi-Breed Evaluation. 2024. Available at: https://www.internationalgeneticso
    lutions.com/site/index.php/multi-breed-genetic-evaluation. [Accessed 19 February
    2024].
50. Retallick KJ, Lu D, Garcia A, et al. 431. Genomic selection in the US: where it has
    been and where it is going?. In: Proceedings of 12th world congress on genetics
    applied to livestock production (WCGALP). The Netherlands: Wageningen Aca-
    demic Publishers; 2022. p. 1795–8. https://doi.org/10.3920/978-90-8686-940-
    4_431.
51. Miller S. Genomic selection in beef cattle creates additional opportunities for em-
    bryo technologies to meet industry needs. Reprod Fertil Dev 2022;35(2):98–105.
    https://doi.org/10.1071/RD22233.
52. NBCEC. NBCEC - national beef cattle education Consortium site - hosted by.
    Iowa State University; 2024. Available at: https://www.nbcec.org/about/mission.
    html. [Accessed 19 February 2024].
53. BIF. Guidelines for uniform beef improvement programs. 2023. Available at:
    https://guidelines.beefimprovement.org/index.php/Guidelines_for_Uniform_Be
    ef_Improvement_Programs. [Accessed 7 July 2023].
54. BIF. Whole Herd Reporting — BIF Guidelines Wiki. 2021. Available at: http://
    guidelines.beefimprovement.org/index.php?title=Whole_Herd_Reporting&oldi
    d=2338.
55. Oliveira HR, Brito LF, Miller SP, et al. Using Random Regression Models to Genet-
    ically Evaluate Functional Longevity Traits in North American Angus Cattle. Ani-
    mals 2020;10(12):2410. https://doi.org/10.3390/ani10122410.
56. Alvarenga AB, Oliveira HR, Turner SP, et al. Unraveling the phenotypic and
    genomic background of behavioral plasticity and temperament in North Amer-
    ican Angus cattle. Genet Sel Evol 2023;55(1):3. https://doi.org/10.1186/s12711-
    023-00777-3.
57. Zoetis. Technical Bulletin: Inherit Select for commercial females. 2022. Available
    at: https://www3.zoetisus.com/animal-genetics/media/documents/inherit/inherit-
    select-technical-bulletin.pdf. [Accessed 19 August 2023].
58. Neogen. Igenity ® Angus Gold Results Key. 2024. Available at: https://www.
    neogen.com/globalassets/pim/assets/original/10018/official_angus-gold_broch
    ure.pdf. [Accessed 19 February 2024].
59. Neogen. Igenity Beef | Genomics | Neogen. 2024. Available at: https://www.
    neogen.com/categories/igenity-profiles/igenity-beef/?recommendationId=317
    6689814511. [Accessed 19 February 2024].
60. Neogen. Igenity+ Envigor. 2024. Available at: https://www.neogen.com/glo
    balassets/pim/assets/original/10000/official_igenity-beef-envigor_brochure.pdf.
    [Accessed 19 February 2024].
61. Neogen. Igenity Feeder | Neogen. 2024. Available at: https://www.neogen.com/
    categories/igenity-profiles/igenity-feeder/?recommendationId=3176689814661.
    [Accessed 19 February 2024].
62. Neogen. Igenity BeefxDairy | Genomics | Neogen. 2024. Available at: https://
    www.neogen.com/categories/igenity-profiles/igenity-beefxdairy/?recommendat
    ionId=3176689814611. [Accessed 19 February 2024].
63. Venegas L, López P, Derome N, et al. Leveraging microbiome information for an-
    imal genetic improvement. Trends Genet 2023;39(10):721–3. https://doi.org/10.
    1016/j.tig.2023.07.004.
64. Pérez-Enciso M, Zingaretti LM, Ramayo-Caldas Y, et al. Opportunities and limits
    of combining microbiome and genome data for complex trait prediction. Genet
    Sel Evol 2021;53(1):65. https://doi.org/10.1186/s12711-021-00658-7.

65. Workman AM, Heaton MP, Vander Ley BL, et al. First gene-edited calf with reduced susceptibility to a major viral pathogen. In: Bartolomei M, editor. PNAS Nexus 2023;2(5):1–14. https://doi.org/10.1093/pnasnexus/pgad125.

66. Clark EL, Archibald AL, Daetwyler HD, et al. From FAANG to fork: application of highly annotated genomes to improve farmed animal production. Genome Biol 2020;21(1):285. https://doi.org/10.1186/s13059-020-02197-8.

67. Koltes JE, Cole JB, Clemmens R, et al. A Vision for Development and Utilization of High-Throughput Phenotyping and Big Data Analytics in Livestock. Front Genet 2019;10:480865. https://doi.org/10.3389/fgene.2019.01197.

68. Christensen OF, Börner V, Varona L, et al. Genetic evaluation including intermediate omics features. Genetics 2021;219(2). https://doi.org/10.1093/genetics/iyab130.

69. Zhao T, Zeng J, Cheng H. Extend mixed models to multilayer neural networks for genomic prediction including intermediate omics data. In: Goddard M, editor. Genetics 2022;221(1). https://doi.org/10.1093/genetics/iyac034.

70. Shirzadifar A, Miar Y, Plastow G, et al. A machine learning approach to predict the most and the least feed–efficient groups in beef cattle. Smart Agric Technol 2023; 5:100317. https://doi.org/10.1016/j.atech.2023.100317.

Future Directions for Ruminant Genomics

Jessica L. Klabnik, DVM, MPH, PhD[a],*, John Dustin Loy, DVM, PhD[b],
Nial J. O'Boyle, BVSc, MS, MBA, MRCVS[c]

KEYWORDS

- Genomics • Testing • Dairy • Beef • Veterinary

KEY POINTS

- Identifying animals that received favorable alleles from parental genetics are crucial for the selection decisions as most economically important traits are genetically complex.
- Genetic selection can be used to enhance animal health and welfare, in addition to increasing economic efficiency.
- Veterinarians can offer invaluable guidance in applying genomic data to improve productivity, health, and economic returns because of their expertise in herd health, genetics, and management.
- Technologies and best practices will continue to evolve at a local level and targets will continue to encourage international collaboration.

INTRODUCTION

This issue of *Veterinary Clinics of North America: Food Animal Practice* was designed to provide both an overview of bovine genetics and genomics and to provide examples for use cases and applications in veterinary practice. Major themes throughout the edition provide background on applications for beef practitioners and dairy practitioners, and also the emerging trends of "beef-on-dairy" practices. This final portion of the edition serves as a forward-looking synopsis to provide animal scientists, beef and dairy producers, veterinary clinicians, reproductive specialists, and genomic scientists with some perspectives and insights into the current state of the industry and some areas where future work may hold additional promise for production gains, identification of genetic diseases, and streamlined breeding and selection approaches framed for the perspective of a practicing bovine clinician.

[a] Department of Clinical Sciences, College of Veterinary Medicine, 1500 Wire Road, Auburn, AL 36830, USA; [b] Nebraska Veterinary Diagnostic Center, School of Veterinary Medicine and Biomedical Sciences, University of Nebraska-Lincoln, 115B NVDC, 4040 East Campus Loop North, Lincoln, NE 68583-0907, USA; [c] School of Veterinary Medicine and Science, University of Nottingham, Sutton Bonington Campus, Leicestershire LE12 5RD, UK
* Corresponding author.
E-mail address: jlk0066@auburn.edu

Vet Clin Food Anim 40 (2024) 459–466
https://doi.org/10.1016/j.cvfa.2024.05.010
0749-0720/24/Published by Elsevier Inc.

UNWAVERING FOUNDATIONS

As highlighted by Troy N. Rowan's article, "Genetics and Genomics 101," in this issue, identifying animals with desired traits and utilizing them as parents for subsequent generations is not a new concept. Methods have developed from purely visual to genomically informed genetic merit estimates, with progressively increasing accuracy. Uncovering DNA, genes, and single nucleotide polymorphisms (SNPs) was just the beginning of understanding the molecular mechanisms underlying inheritance. Traits with simple inheritance patterns, such as polledness and certain congenital genetic defects, are readily testable and allow for managed mating of carriers.[1,2] This allows producers to maximize genetic diversity and reduce unnecessary culling of carrier animals. Unfortunately, many economic traits are complex, driven by hundreds or thousands of causal mutations. Complex traits are harder to predict from parental phenotypes, therefore identifying animals that received favorable bits of parental genetics is crucial for the selection decisions. Selection accuracy and generation interval are the main drivers of genetic progress.

Estimated breeding values (EBVs) are the statistical estimate of an animal's genetic potential and can be utilized to improve selection accuracy and, when paired with advanced reproductive technologies, reduce generational interval. Calculation of EBVs is typically performed by breed associations or other third-party organizations. In the dairy and beef industries, these are typically reported as predicted transmitting abilities and estimated progeny differences (EPDs) respectfully. These can be calculated for any heritable trait in which enough phenotypes are recorded, but their accuracy can be greatly enhanced by the inclusion of genomics. Genomic enhancement requires analyzing a large set of molecular markers and statistically analyzing their relationship and probabilities of getting inherited together. Tests to analyze these markers utilize microarray technologies; the more variants assayed, the more accurate the predictors. Commonly, 20,000 to 100,000 variants are assayed. Elite sires can be identified at a younger age through genomically enhanced EBVs, compared to waiting until they sire offspring.

BEEF GENETIC EVALUATIONS AND GENOMICS

Matthew L. Spangler and Donagh P. Berry's article, "Beef Genetic Evaluations," in this issue provide an overview of classic and routine genetic evaluations and the evolution these evaluations have undertaken in the last 50 years of practice and application.[3] The early foundations of this work relied primarily on visual assessment but transitioned into quantitative traits using data and phenotypes that are straightforward to measure. The number and types of traits evaluated have expanded significantly, and thus the importance of accurate phenotypes has also become more significant as the diversity of phenotypes that are now possible to collect has increased. The investigators highlight traits such as methane emissions and carcass ultrasound, as some that have been enabled by advances in technology. Additionally, as more and more traits become "phenotypeable" and available for selection, this has led to the development of indexes that combine multiple traits that should align with the goals of the breeder.

The advent of genomics provided initial challenges with commercial companies delivering metrics to rank animals on genomic tests, which had mixed results. One of the core developments using different statistical models has been the implementation of genomics to enhance the accuracy of EBVs, where for some breeds genomic supplementation of EBVs allows for predictions with the same level of accuracy as if there were 5 to 25 offspring, allowing for much more rapid genetic progress. It should be noted that many of these are breed/geographically specific and care should be taken in applying these values to animals outside of the population used to calculate them. Additionally, they remind us that economic selection indexes are case dependent and breeding objectives need to inform the index and how it is developed. The investigators provide an examination of economic indexes for producers that retain all animals through the market versus those that only retain replacement females. The traits that support terminal markets (carcass, marbling, rate of gain) are much different from those for replacement heifers (longevity, cow cost, calving ease), and are often antagonistic. Therefore, matching indexes with the goals of the producers is extremely important to maximize economic benefits.

Genetic selection can be used to enhance animal health and welfare. One example involving calving difficulties is illustrated in Susanne Hinkley and Rich G. Tait's article, "Sampling and Laboratory Logistics: How to Collect DNA Samples and Overview of Techniques for Laboratory Analysis," in this issue, by Dr Mueller, Dr Courter, and Dr Spare. Dystocias have an immediate and prolonged impact on animal health and herd economics. Incorporating genetic selection for calving ease traits, such as selecting for balanced calving ease direct or maternal calving ease, reduces the prevalence of dystocia. In the case example in which producers worked with veterinarians to select for relevant EBVs, dystocia was reduced from 35% to less than 1% and coinciding calf mortality was also reduced, providing measurable and valuable economic and health and welfare impacts to the animals and animal health providers. Veterinarians with working knowledge of EBVs can assist producers with the selection of animals that meet the herd goals. Traditionally, EBVs were only available as seed stock to producers. However, with advancing genomic technology, commercial producers will also be able to genetically select in an intentional, comprehensive way to meet their production goals.

Genomic technology is proven to enhance profitability, but uptake has lagged behind other production animal sectors.[4] The investigators highlight 3 levels of investment that can be utilized differently based on the producer's role in the beef supply chain. These levels include parentage verification, genomically enhanced EPDs, and commercial genomic testing. Parentage verification can add value in a variety of scenarios, including ensuring animals are marketed accurately and determining parentage in herds that use multi-sire pastures. Genomically enhanced EPDs provide the most accurate predictions of genetic merit and can be determined at a younger age than traditional methods, allowing for more rapid genetic progress. Because genomically enhanced EPDs are more reliable than traditional EPDs, the breeding outcome is more predictable, and therefore can add value throughout the beef industry. Commercial genomic testing first became available in the early 2000s and has since undergone significant advancements and improvements. Two options exist: firstly, generating commercial EPDs by reporting pedigrees and phenotypes to a genetic evaluation provider, and secondly, submitting DNA samples to obtain estimates solely from the animal's genetic makeup. These promising tools are underutilized, and continued research for improving accuracy and subsequent validation will be critical for further implementation. Undoubtable, genomic information will continue to be integrated throughout beef production systems, resulting in increased efficiency and profitability as they become further aligned with the needs and goals of the production systems.

GENOMIC TECHNOLOGIES—SAMPLING AND LABORATORY TESTING

In order to enable genomic-based selection, a fundamental requirement is the acquisition of high-quality genomics data from the animals of interest. Maci L. Mueller and colleagues' article, "Innovating Beef Cattle Veterinary Practices: Leveraging Genetic and Genomic Tools," in this issue provide a thorough overview of the proper methods for sample collection and submission, and an overview of the methods used to generate genomic data. They provide an overview and best practices for use of common collection devices, such as tissue sampling technologies or tissue sampling units, which frequently offer barcoded unique identification.[5] Additionally, they provide some clarification on the diverse types of "genotyping" that are available through testing and include parentage analysis, screening for recessive conditions, and/or evaluation of economically important genetic markers such as SNPs.[6] Recommendations on postmortem sample collection are also provided that enable preservation of potential genetic information that may be required for future investigations. Typically, this includes the collection of skin or muscle followed by prompt freezing to halt decomposition to ensure effective testing in the future. Other tissues undergo DNA degradation at differing intervals, and those, such as organs, may also be contaminated with higher levels of postmortem overgrowth of bacteria that can interfere with testing, so these tissue types are less favored for collection.[7] Finally, the investigators stress that proper sample identification is critical to ensure accuracy allowing for full utilization of testing results. Improper or mislabeled identification can quickly make the whole testing process futile, and lead to inaccurate or improper selection decisions or provide misleading data to breed associations or others that rely on it.

THE ROLE OF PRACTITIONERS

Patrick M.R. Comyn's article, "The Private Practitioner: A Veterinary Practitioner's Perspective to the Application of Bovine Genomics in Client Herds"; and Kim Egan's article, "Role of Veterinary Practitioners in the Genomic Era in Dairy – Economic Impact," in this issue illustrate how veterinary practitioners are uniquely positioned to integrate genomic technologies into both dairy and beef cattle operations. By leveraging their expertise in herd health, genetics, and management, veterinarians can offer invaluable guidance in applying genomic data to improve productivity, health, and economic returns. Dr Kim Egan and Dr Patrick Comyn highlight the transformative potential of genomics, showing how veterinarians can optimize breeding strategies, enhance disease resistance, and increase overall efficiency in dairy and beef herds.

Patrick M.R. Comyn's article, "The Private Practitioner: A Veterinary Practitioner's Perspective to the Application of Bovine Genomics in Client Herds," in this issue emphasizes the significant impact of genomic technologies on the beef industry. Genomic evaluation allows for precise selection of economically important traits, such as carcass characteristics, feed efficiency, and reproductive performance, thereby improving expected progeny differences. This precision has driven the beef-on-dairy phenomenon, where beef sires are used on dairy cows to produce crossbred calves with higher market value due to improved meat quality and yield. For example, Angus sires with high calving ease and low-birth-weight expected progeny differences are favored to minimize calving difficulties while enhancing growth traits like weaning weight. The adoption of genomic screening has expanded the population of evaluated bulls, allowing for more robust selection and accelerated genetic improvements.

Veterinarians play a crucial role in this genomic revolution by educating clients about the impact of genomic testing on animal health and productivity, integrating genomic data with existing production metrics, and supporting reproductive management through the application of gender-sorted semen and beef-on-dairy strategies. They provide decision-making assistance, helping clients select sires and dams based on genomic evaluations to achieve desired traits and manage environmental factors that influence gene expression and animal performance.

Kim Egan's article, "Role of Veterinary Practitioners in the Genomic Era in Dairy – Economic Impact," in this issue examines the economic benefits of using genetic data to enhance profitability in dairy and beef herds. Genomic testing significantly improves milk yield and overall herd health by identifying cows with superior genetic potential for milk production and disease resistance. This enables producers to focus breeding efforts on high-potential cows, enhancing herd performance and reducing veterinary costs. For instance, genomic testing can identify cows with higher genetic merit for traits such as milk production and daughter pregnancy rate (DPR). By selecting cows with high DPR, producers can increase conception rates and overall reproductive performance, leading to a higher percentage of cows reaching peak milk production.

High fertility levels also enable the use of advanced reproductive techniques, such as sexed semen, further enhancing the genetic quality of the herd. Genomic evaluations facilitate the early identification of high-value animals, accelerating genetic progress by reducing generational intervals. This early selection shortens the generational interval, enabling quicker improvements in herd genetics and productivity. Improving feed efficiency is another critical benefit of genomic testing; by identifying cows that convert feed into milk more efficiently, producers can optimize feed use and reduce costs. Given that feed costs typically constitute over half of total expenses, improvements in feed efficiency can have a substantial economic impact. Additionally, genomic data assist in improving overall herd health by identifying cows with genetic predispositions to health conditions, allowing producers to implement targeted management practices.

Looking forward, Dr Kim Egan and Dr Comyn highlight the significant future applications of genomics in dairy and beef cattle operations. Dr Egan emphasizes that future genomic technologies will enable detailed genome analyses, identifying genetic predispositions to various health conditions and allowing for the development of more effective preventative measures and treatments. This will enhance overall herd health and reduce the need for costly veterinary interventions. Dr Egan also foresees advancements in robotic milking systems, where genomic data will help breed cows with traits optimized for automated environments, such as moderate body size and ideal teat placement, thus improving efficiency and productivity in dairy operations.

Dr Comyn discusses the future of genomic applications in the beef industry, particularly through low-pass whole genome sequencing. This technology will allow for a much more comprehensive analysis of genetic traits, identifying factors such as susceptibility to disease, which are currently difficult to assess using current methods. Additionally, Dr Comyn anticipates the integration of carcass merit data into genomic predictions, driven by the beef-on-dairy strategy. This will result in crossbred calves with enhanced meat quality, which will become more valuable in the market and increase returns for producers that implement such a strategy. Moreover, the use of advanced reproductive techniques like in vitro fertilization and embryo transfer, coupled with genomic data, will enable the propagation of high-value genetics more efficiently, thus accelerating genetic progress in beef herds.

Both Dr Egan and Dr Comyn stress the critical role of veterinarians in these advancements, guiding producers to leverage genomic data for optimizing breeding strategies, improving animal health, and enhancing overall productivity. By staying at the forefront of genomic innovations, veterinarians can ensure that both dairy and beef operations achieve significant future production gains and economic benefits.

INTERNATIONAL AND NATIONAL GENOMICS

The Marco Winters and colleagues' article, "European Dairy Cattle Evaluations and International Use of Genomic Data"; and Donagh P. Berry and Matthew L. Spangler's article, "The Benefit of a National Genomic Testing Scheme," in this issue illustrate the critical roles of both international collaborations and national genotyping initiatives in genetic advancement, along with the challenges and opportunities in their implementation. Platforms like Interbull and EuroGenomics, as discussed by Winters, are pivotal in pooling global phenotypic and genomic data. This collaboration improves the accuracy of breeding values and allows farmers to make informed breeding decisions based on an extensive genetic database, fostering sustainable livestock management practices.

Building on the global perspective, Donagh P. Berry and Matthew L. Spangler's article, "The Benefit of a National Genomic Testing Scheme," in this issue transitions to the national scale, emphasizing how genotyping programs within countries empower precise management of genetic resources. These programs enable effective tracking of animal pedigrees, health traits, and productivity characteristics, which are vital for managing genetic diversity and preventing inbreeding—key factors in maintaining long-term livestock productivity and health. National genotyping initiatives provide complete traceability from birth to slaughter, enhancing food safety and marketability. Additionally, they facilitate parentage verification, significantly reducing errors and improving the accuracy of genetic evaluations. This comprehensive approach ensures that individual animals' genetic merit can be accurately assessed, supporting better-informed breeding and management decisions.

Navigating the balance between open data exchange and the protection of commercial interests remains a challenge. Ensuring the continued success of genomic initiatives requires fostering collaborative environments that encourage sharing and innovation. Building on the collaborative frameworks highlighted by both Winters and Berry, the integration of advanced genomic tools such as SNP chips, next-generation sequencing, and machine learning algorithms will further empower these partnerships. These technologies enable the precise analysis and management of vast genetic datasets, enhancing both the speed and accuracy of genetic evaluations. By utilizing these tools, international and national collaborations can streamline data-sharing processes, optimize breeding strategies, and accelerate sustainable genetic advancements in the livestock sector. Both articles highlight how national and international genomic initiatives support environmental targets: nationally, by optimizing local resources and improving production efficiencies tailored to specific regional needs. Technologies and best practices will continue to evolve at a local level[8,9] and targets will continue to encourage international collaboration.[10]

ADVANCING GENETICS WITH GENOMIC TECHNOLOGY

Without doubt, cattle industries have advanced in sustainability and productivity by utilizing technological advances. Dr Diniz and Dr Banerjee highlight technological advances in the dairy and beef industries in Priyanka Banerjee and Wellison J.S. Diniz's article, "Advancing Dairy and Beef Genetics Through Genomic Technologies," in this issue. These include targeting novel traits, genome editing, and high-throughput phenotyping. Novel traits such as efficiency, longevity, health, fertility, temperament, and conformation are important to both industries. Collecting phenotypes associated with these traits has classically been challenging, but recent advances in technology have allowed for novel methods to generate data for selection. For example, fertility, which is a lowly heritable trait, has been a challenge in the dairy industry. Research into utilizing mid-infrared spectroscopy (MFERT: fertility predicted using mid-infrared spectroscopy) and reproductive tract size and position score as phenotypes may improve our ability to genomically select cows with higher fertility.[11,12] Similarly, immune response traits may impact mastitis incidence. Another example would be selecting for feed-efficient cattle with reduced methane emission.[10] In the beef industry, cow efficiency and sustainability are of great interest, as feed and replacement costs are large drivers of production costs in cow-calf operations. The investigators provided a table of commercially available genomic tests for beef cattle that evaluate many different traits and economic indexes. Several groups, such as the National Cattle Evaluation Consortium and Beef Improvement Federation, are striving to provide guidelines and standardize genetic evaluations for the improvement of the national beef herd.

Research involving genome editing and high-throughput phenotyping demonstrates possible advances in understanding complex traits and the possibility of new tools to genetically improve cattle. Understanding the interactions between genomics, transcriptomics, proteomics, metabolomics, and epigenomics will further our ability to predict and capitalize on functional changes resulting from differing treatments or management decisions. Genome editing through the clustered regularly interspaced short palindromic repeats (CRISPR)-cas9 system has already successfully produced cattle with economically relevant traits, such as bovine vial diarrhea virus resistance and polledness.[13] Emerging opportunities to improve these technologies are expected and may include sensors, intermediate omics features, multilayer neural networks, and machine learning.

SUMMARY

The integration of genomics into the dairy and beef industries is multifaceted. Selection of superior sires, selection of superior dams, and parentage testing are readily incorporated. The use of genomic analysis to identify animals with lowly heritable traits and the development of new traits will continue to increase in demand. Veterinarians play a crucial role by educating clients, integrating genomic data with existing metrics, and assisting in decision-making that will impact the future shape of the global herd.

CLINICS CARE POINTS

- Selection of complex traits requires continued sophistication and application of technologies and breeding values to support continued improvement.
- The development of indexes to help select for multiple traits is beneficial, but the traits should be aligned with the goals of the producer.
- With increasing use of technologies such as low-pass whole genome sequencing, the collection and proper identification of high-quality samples are critical.
- By leveraging their expertise in herd health, genetics, and management, veterinarians can offer invaluable guidance in applying genomic data to improve productivity, health, and economic returns.

DISCLOSURE

The authors have nothing to disclose.

REFERENCES

1. Wiedemar N, Tetens J, Jagannathan V, et al. Independent Polled Mutations Leading to Complex Gene Expression Differences in Cattle. PLoS One 2014;9(3): e93435. https://doi.org/10.1371/journal.pone.0093435.
2. Cieploch A, Rutkowska K, Oprzadek J, et al. Genetic disorders in beef cattle: a review. Genes Genomics 2017;39(5):461–71. https://doi.org/10.1007/s13258-017-0525-8.
3. Golden BL, Garrick DJ, Benyshek LL. Milestones in beef cattle genetic evaluation. J Anim Sci 2009;87(14 Suppl):E3–10. https://doi.org/10.2527/jas.2008-1430.
4. Rolf MM, Decker JE, McKay SD, et al. Genomics in the United States beef industry. Livestock Sci 2014;166:84–93. https://doi.org/10.1016/j.livsci.2014.06.005.
5. de Groot M, Ras T, van Haeringen WA. Application of allflex conservation buffer in illumina genotyping1. J Anim Sci 2016;94(12):5023–7. https://doi.org/10.2527/jas.2016-0855.
6. Wiggans GR, Cole JB, Hubbard SM, et al. Genomic Selection in Dairy Cattle: The USDA Experience. Annu Rev Anim Biosci 2017;5:309–27. https://doi.org/10.1146/annurev-animal-021815-111422.
7. Tozzo P, Scrivano S, Sanavio M, et al. The Role of DNA Degradation in the Estimation of Post-Mortem Interval: A Systematic Review of the Current Literature. Int J Mol Sci 2020;21(10). https://doi.org/10.3390/ijms21103540.
8. McParland S, Frizzarin M, Lahart B, et al. Predicting methane emissions of individual grazing dairy cows from spectral analyses of their milk samples. J Dairy Sci 2024;107(2):978–91. https://doi.org/10.3168/jds.2023-23577.
9. Winters M, Coffey M. The EnviroCow index and its impact on the UK dairy industry's carbon footprint. Paper presented at: 2023 Interbull Annual meeting will be held at CENTRE DE CONGRÈS DE LYON, 50 Quai Charles de Gaulle, 69006 Lyon, France from 26-27 August, 2023; Lyon, France.
10. van Staaveren N, Rojas de Oliveira H, Houlahan K, et al. The Resilient Dairy Genome Project-A general overview of methods and objectives related to feed efficiency and methane emissions. J Dairy Sci 2024;107(3):1510–22. https://doi.org/10.3168/jds.2022-22951.
11. Martin AAA, de Oliveira G Jr, Madureira AML, et al. Reproductive tract size and position score: Estimation of genetic parameters for a novel fertility trait in dairy cows. J Dairy Sci 2022;105(10):8189–98. https://doi.org/10.3168/jds.2021-21651.
12. Van den Berg I, Stephen M, Ho P, et al. New phenotypes for genetic improvement of fertility in dairy cows. In: Hermesch S, Dominik S, editors. Breeding focus 2021 - improving reproduction. Armidale (Australia): Animal Genetics and Breeding Unit; 2021. p. 59–70.
13. Workman AM, Heaton MP, Vander Ley BL, et al. First gene-edited calf with reduced susceptibility to a major viral pathogen. PNAS Nexus 2023;2(5):pgad125. https://doi.org/10.1093/pnasnexus/pgad125.

Moving?

Make sure your subscription moves with you!

To notify us of your new address, find your **Clinics Account Number** (located on your mailing label above your name), and contact customer service at:

Email: journalscustomerservice-usa@elsevier.com

800-654-2452 (subscribers in the U.S. & Canada)
314-447-8871 (subscribers outside of the U.S. & Canada)

Fax number: 314-447-8029

Elsevier Health Sciences Division
Subscription Customer Service
3251 Riverport Lane
Maryland Heights, MO 63043

*To ensure uninterrupted delivery of your subscription, please notify us at least 4 weeks in advance of move.

Printed and bound by CPI Group (UK) Ltd, Croydon, CR0 4YY

08/05/2025

01864724-0008

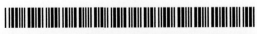